From Co

A Guide to Navigating Cancer in Your 30's

By: Meredith Goldberg

Thanks for not firing me for writing this -haha ☺

Dedication

For the Jeanster and El Jeffe

Preface

On August 18, 2010, I was diagnosed with Focal Ductal Carcinoma In-Situ (DCIS) breast cancer in my left breast. To this day, I'm still not sure that the entire experience has really hit me. I was 32 and had never had surgery; I'd never even had a cavity, so you can imagine my shock when I got a call from my nurse practitioner asking me if I was alone or at work.

Cancer. Awesome.

What followed was more than a year and a half of MRIs, visits to plastic surgeons and oncologists, surgery, chemotherapy and radiation, all while most of my friends were getting married and having kids. Quite the spectrum of rites of passage. So what do you do besides cry and scream when all you want to do is be like everyone else, but that's just not in the cards for you? Well, that's what this book is for. Unwillingly I suppose, I became the guinea pig for all of my friends when it came to knowing the ins and outs of having breast cancer. What started as an informal way of trying to keep my friends in the loop with what was happening each step of the way on my journey became this book—a chronological account of my life and the crazy, ridiculous, scary and lifesaving events that followed.

As soon as I was diagnosed, I hightailed it to the health and wellness section at my local chain bookstore. "Surely there's a book for this," I thought to myself. "Surely someone in my age range has gone through this already and has some insight to lend, foods to eat, things to do, music to listen to." I wanted reassurance and some sense of solidarity. I was looking for anything to know that I wasn't alone.

Nothing. There was nothing for a fairly well-adjusted, educated, sarcastic and pissed off woman whose life had just been uprooted. My friends wanted me to keep a blog, "You're funny. You should start a blog," they'd say. But I didn't want to. I wanted to deal with the disease head-on and move on, but the further I became entrenched in the day-to-day dealings with the disease, and as more friends and family found out about my illness through the grapevine, the more they wanted to know. And the truth is that I didn't mind talking about it. In fact, I found that when talking about what was going on with friends and family, I'd feel better. I took to my laptop on nights I couldn't sleep from a mix of anxiety and the steroids I was forced to take the day before, of and after chemotherapy sessions. I'd write email updates once every three weeks or so to let everyone know that I was still here, still joking and being "myself." I wanted everyone to know that this disease was not going to claim me. I would send updates about my hilarious run-ins with nurses, about the crazy hair-freezing therapy I was trying to conserve my hair during chemo and funny things my parents did when they were staying with me in Washington DC. Every once in a while, I'd open up and let them know how scared I was, and how uncomfortable the process really was as much as I joked about everyday minutiae.

Those emails were a great form of therapy for me, so I've chosen to include some of them at the beginning of each chapter.

The unfortunate truth is that many people are going to go through what I went through, or at least something like it. And I'd hazard the guess that many of you won't want to read about how free and amazing you will feel once you shave your head or how a prayer circle or wearing a ton of pink will cure you of your anxieties. (Not that I have anything against pink). Regardless of the kind of cancer you have just been handed, you probably will feel something similar to what I felt after being diagnosed—a basic desire to feel like other people were out there with me. And let's face it, most practical people need a guide book to navigate the scary, painful and even at times hilarious events that will occur as you battle this evil and cruel disease.

  In 2015, it was reported that about 231,840 new cases of invasive breast cancer will be diagnosed in women; about 60,290 new cases of carcinoma in situ (CIS) will be diagnosed (CIS is non-invasive and is the earliest form of breast cancer) and about 40,290 women will die from breast cancer. I am grateful to be a survivor, but looking at these numbers as a woman is not an easy thing to do. So in a way, I'm glad that my experience encouraged me to arm myself with all of this knowledge. And now I can share it with you.

  Breast cancer is the second leading cause of cancer death in women, exceeded only by lung cancer. The chance that breast cancer will be responsible for a woman's death is about 1 in 36 (about 3%). After increasing for more than two decades, female breast cancer incidence rates began decreasing in 2000, then dropped by about 7% from 2002 to 2003. This large decrease was thought to be due to the decline in use of hormone therapy after menopause that occurred after the results of the Women's Health Initiative were published in 2002.

Thankfully, death rates from breast cancer have been declining since about 1989, with larger decreases in women younger than 50. There's obviously better technology out there for treatment as research progresses, which is commonly cited as a probably reason for these decreases. They're also believed to be the result of earlier detection through screening and increased awareness, which is another reason why I'm writing this I guess. The more aware we all are, the better. Incidence rates of in situ breast cancer rose rapidly during the 1980s and 1990s largely because of increases in mammography screening, meaning that the more that doctors and the general public know about breast cancer, the more they're finding it and the more we are trying to kick its ass.[1]

So, this book is for you. Young women who are practical. Those who are lost in a sea of path reports and films. Those who cannot fathom the fact that cancer is cured by yoga. Those that don't want to sit in the circle of trust and share their stories. While my particular experience was with breast cancer, I feel like there's something in here for everyone dealing with a scary diagnosis—from how to find a great surgeon to figuring out what foods might make you feel better. You may just want to know that you aren't alone in your day-to-day dealings with a ridiculous situation.

While it may seem like the end of the world, cancer for many, is not, and as my best friend rationalized it, "At least you don't have herpes, that shit is for life"

So true, my friends, so true.

I've chosen to share my journey so you can witness my ups and downs of dealing with this disease; sometimes you're not going to have the best day and the recipient of your rage could be your doctor, a parent or a friend. I had days where as much as I knew that my doctors were only trying to help, they were met with resistance and resentment—feelings that I know were about the situation, not things my doctors did or didn't do. More often than not, I felt bad immediately about my misplaced rage, but fortunately anger wasn't a constant for me. I also had days where I felt forever grateful for the group of friends and family that helped me to rally and fight the disease with every inch of my being. I'm not a saint, I never claimed to be, but I'm hardly a sinner, just some girl who got blindsided by a disease that in 2011, an estimated 230,480 other women were blindsided with.[2]

It's OK to laugh, it's OK to make light of it, it's OK to have a glass of wine with good friends and sneak a cigarette, it's OK to sit in the sun at the beach sometimes and it's OK to be so angry that you tell your mother to fuck off and then burst into tears and then call and apologize and get mad all over again.

It's not fun, it's not easy and when you're young, it's a major lifestyle change. But, it's doable, I promise.

Chapter 1: My Story (March 2010- August 18, 2010)

I've dubbed the summer of 2010 "my summer of yes." And it didn't take me much retrospection to give it such a title. Right after emerging from a three year relationship (that lasted about a year longer than it should have) in March, I was relieved to be alone and spend the spring and summer months reclaiming a life that had gotten a little away from me over the course of my relationship.

Step #1: Book a ticket to a college friend's wedding in Greece that July with some of my closest friends. A long weekend in Corfu, followed by a week in Preveza, Greece for a once in a lifetime opportunity to be a part of an actual "Big Fat Greek Wedding." There was no chance I was going to miss it.

Step #2: Find a new job. After finally finishing my masters earlier that year, I was determined to take my new degree in Marketing and find myself a job that didn't involve press releases about HVAC units and standby generators. I wanted to rid myself of clients who didn't care about the work I did. I was ready to sink my teeth into what would become a career. Finding a job in the summer of 2010 in the economic state was no small feat, and I had finally found an opportunity that seemed to be a great fit for exactly what I wanted to do.

Step #3: Date. After getting out of a destructive relationship, I needed to shake off some of the damage that had been done on both sides, I remember waking up on my friend's couch the morning after my ex-fiancé and I had finally ended things. I felt refreshed and relieved and ready to enjoy being alone again. I had my apartment back to myself, I slept in the middle of the bed, I ate peanut butter and jelly straight from the jar with a spoon while I sat on my couch and watched endless hours of terrible television. I went out on Tuesdays and flirted with strangers, slowly gaining back the confidence that had been taken from me for the last six months of my stale relationship. I wasn't necessarily ready to date seriously, but I wanted to have fun, meet new people, and let's be honest: I was ready for a great one-night-stand.

In mid-July, about a week before my Greek adventure, I felt something weird happened that momentarily jostled me out of my new routine. As I was getting into bed, I rolled over onto my stomach and felt something towards the top of my left breast. At the time, I could only explain the sensation to myself as a pulled muscle since it hurt most acutely when I rolled over onto it and was located closer to my sternum. "That feels weird," I thought to myself as I shrugged it off and slowly faded into a deep sleep. When I woke up the next morning and it was still there, so I did what every woman with non-refundable tickets to Greece would do: I ignored it. "I've been working out a lot, it must just be a pulled muscle," I rationalized as I packed my suitcase. And off I went on my trip and had some of the most memorable trip ever with some of my best college friends. During those ten days, I laughed until I couldn't breathe, I drank semi-fredos and smoked unfiltered cigarettes for breakfast; I ate fried mullet, drank white wine and smoked more unfiltered cigarettes for dinner. I had, at this point, been restored to my former carefree, easy-going, light-hearted self.

But every now and then during those ten days, I'd feel it; that oddly shaped bump on my left breast. I felt it while lying on the beach, while watching my friends get married; it was there and it wasn't going away. About a week after being home, I finally told a friend "Hey, I have this bump that won't go away, feel this" to which they said, "Just go get it checked out. Don't be lazy about it". I did, and that's when the fun really began.

I called my gynecologist, since she had been the one who had been giving my boobs the obligatory squeeze since I had started seeing her during college. She told me to come right in and even though she wasn't available to see me, a nurse practitioner in the office would be able to examine me. I feel what you're talking about," she told me, "But it doesn't feel like anything serious. It seems like a fatty mass—but I'd like for you to have a sonogram done, just so we can be sure."

She wasn't worried, so why should I worry? This was the attitude I had going into my first sonogram. Since I "knew" it was nothing, I had gone alone and hadn't told many people; I hadn't even told my mother w has been known, at times, to overreact (I have a Jewish mother from Long Island, you do the math).

So off I went, into the sonogram room with the technician. She explained what she was going to do as I looked at my watch. I had taken a Friday off of work for the appointment and was antsy to do other errands as long I was off work. I had to go to the bank and was meeting a friend for lunch and I needed a manicure—all of those typical single-30-something things to do. As the technician ran the sonogram across my chest, I looked up at the monitor and saw it: an oddly shaped dark spot towards the left side of my left breast, nowhere near my "fatty mass." Immediately, I could feel my stomach drop. All women (and men, for that matter) have gut feelings—like when you just know that someone's lying to you, or that he didn't just forget to call. That kind of sinking, inescapable gut feeling. As if she were responding to my building anxiety, the technician interrupted my ruminations: "I need to have the radiologist look at the results and I think we'll need to do a mammogram to get more information."

I burst into tears immediately.

There I was, missing my manicure to get my very first mammogram. Most doctors recommend that women get their first mammogram at 35, yet there I was at 32, three years early, getting my breasts smooshed in a laundry press—a cold plastic slab attached to a monstrous white metal arm that looked like it belonged in a top secret facility rather than on in a downtown DC doctor's office. In addition to the fact that the machine itself couldn't have been more unwelcoming, the room was ice cold and my cotton gown was not doing much to help the chills that were running through my entire body. And the mammogram process itself is not fun: it feels like a weight is being dropped on top of you—and when you aren't really sure why you're getting one in the first place, it's even scarier.

The experience that followed my mammogram was possibly one of the worst interactions that I've ever had with another human being, the radiologist. Here is the job of a radiologist, "A radiologist is a medical doctor that uses technology, computers, medical imaging and medical equipment like MRI, computed tomography (CT Scans), and ultrasound to assist other doctors in figuring out issues related to their patients' medical conditions." Please note, this description does *not* say, "A radiologist is a medical doctor that can immediately tell you what a small mass the size of your fingertip is or what you should do about it."

And yet the radiologist who I was called into see after my mammogram wasn't terribly nuanced in how she approached the topic of my test results. A tall and narrow woman with an angular and angry face called me into her office and said, point blank, "This looks bad, I'm pretty sure you have cancer." Then, it started to feel like senseless words were coming out of her math. To be honest, I had stopped listening as she rambled on, telling me what my test meant and what I needed to do about it.

As she continued talking, I stared at her small brown eyes and poorly-dyed auburn hair, then up at the light board where my charts were being illuminated, then back at her, then back up at the light board. I was trying to maintain a level of composure that had flown out the window about two hours earlier. My pulled muscle had, in a matter of minutes, turned into cancer. How do does one wrap their head around this drastic turn of events? My mind raced, my palms had grown sweaty and cold, my entire body felt like I had the flu. Unable to comprehend what the radiologist was actually saying, and frankly not in the mood to try, I felt myself go into survival mode. This state was familiar to me: when I feel threatened,

I tend to grow defensive and combative, which I have always found to be amusing since it's so far off from my general demeanor. I like to compare myself to a turtle: whenever I feel any sort of fear, I retreat underneath an armor of terrible behavior.

The radiologist's terrible bedside manner caused me to blurt out some things I'm not terribly proud of. Note: I do not condone saying what follows to any physician, or any person, for that matter, but if you are an intelligent person being told that you have cancer by a woman who has zero authority to do so, you might have said the same. What I said was something along the lines of this:

"STOP! Shut up and stop talking so fast. Who the hell do you think you are, talking to me like that?"

Unphased by my outburst, the radiologist didn't acknowledge my state of panic and instead took my plea for her to stop talking so fast literally. She repeated exactly what she had said to me initially, but a little bit more slowly this time. Of course, I had heard her loud and clear the first time: take my films to my gynecologist, schedule an appointment to get the mass biopsied, and figure out for sure what I was dealing with. I was shocked by her lack of bedside manner. How could people be trained to look for potential cancerous tumors, yet have no idea how to speak to someone that should legitimately be concerned? I stood up, tears streaming down my face, nose running uncontrollably, grabbed the films out of her hand, proclaimed, "I'm too young for this shit." as I walked out the door, down the hallway to my gynecologist's office which was a typical Friday afternoon zoo. I stormed in, stomping past the row of pregnant women who were waiting for their check-ups, past the expectant fathers playing on their phones and right up to the receptionists who were casually chatting. They stopped when I slammed my giant folder containing my films on the desk.

"I need to see a doctor. Now," I said.

Taking one look at my tear-stained face, my runny nose and my shaky hands, the receptionists looked like they felt sorry for me and asked for more information about what was going on. I explained what had just happened, they looked at each other and immediately picked up the phone so I could bypass the line and get in to see the same nurse practitioner that I had seen just days earlier.

"Pulled muscle, huh," I joked with her as she looked at my films. I was trying to shake off the conversation with the radiologist and convince myself that I was fine and had already been plotting how to slash her tires.

"It will be OK," the practitioner said, trying to calm me down. "You'll need to go to Georgetown University Hospital and get a biopsy and then we'll know more."

"So let's go." I replied. At the time, I didn't understand that I was about to embark on a process that, in all honesty, never ends. There's a rhyme and a reason and a method to dealing with cancer, and at that point, I had no idea what any of it was. Specifically, I didn't understand why any waiting would be involved. To most people, the word "cancer" brings with it a sense of urgency. So naturally I assumed that anything having to do with my potential treatment would need to happen at warp speed. I was wrong.

"You'll have to call them and make an appointment," the nurse practitioner explained as she wrote down the numbers of the people that I would need to call, which I did as soon as I walked out of my doctor's office and had a biopsy scheduled for that Wednesday. I had at least five days before I knew what was actually going on with my body. Five days of not knowing. Five days of wondering. Five days without answers. This was possibly one of most helpless days I'd ever had up until that point in my 32 years. So I did what any crazed woman would do who was just told that they probably have cancer: I ran home to my parents' house on Long Island. I had gone straight from the gynecologist's office, back to my apartment, threw clothing in a bag, hopped in a cab, barked "Union Station, please" at the cab driver and was on my way home. I hadn't even told my parents I was coming. Once I was in the cab, I called my mother.

"I'm sick," I bawled into the phone

"WHAT? Meredith I can't hear you. I'm in the car," she yelled back. My mother hasn't exactly mastered the cell phone and I usually refuse to speak to her while she's driving because she hasn't yet grasped the fact that driving and talking is not only illegal, but also extremely dangerous for someone who doesn't drive (or use cell phones) that fluently to begin with. I imagined her sitting behind the wheel of her Honda Civic, Howard Stern blaring through the speakers, cradling the phone as she navigated the streets of Long Island.

Since I hadn't told her or my father anything up until this point, I had a lot of explaining to do, which is hard to do when you're choking back sobs in the backseat of a cab.

By the time I had successfully spit out all my updates of personal turmoil, I was expecting my mother to be in hysterics. But instead, she was calm.

"It's nothing Meredith. Don't get all excited. We'll get it biopsied, and it'll be nothing. I had a mass in my 50s and it was fine. There's no history of it in our family."

All four of my grandparents had already passed away, but none from cancer. Plus, none of the women in my family had ever been diagnosed with breast or ovarian cancer, so genealogy couldn't be the culprit. My mother's attempt to reassure me was valiant, but I still wasn't convinced that I should feel especially "relieved."

I was confused as to why my mother wasn't flying into freak-out mode, since she usually thinks everything is a big deal (and especially things related to my well-being, since I am their only child). Was I the one overreacting? Was my situation really no big deal?

When I finally made it to Long Island, I walked down the steps of the Long Island Rail Road and saw that both her and my father were waiting for me. At that point, I knew that my cause for alarm wasn't unwarranted, since my father is a creature of habit and hates to uproot his routine. He's probably the smartest person I know even though he dresses like a homeless person, hates to leave the house, and refuses to learn how to use a computer. He is a retired teacher and reads in his office for most of the day, every day. So to see that he was in the front seat of the car, rather than at home reading while my mom came and picked me up, felt like a gesture. Once again, I felt validated that my situation was, in fact, a big deal and I wasn't the only one who was scared.

We spent the weekend doing things to forget. We went to the local driving range to hit some golf balls, a hobby that both my mother and father were easing into now that both were retired. We ate lots of bread, which is both my father's and my favorite food of all time. (My mother hasn't touched a carbohydrate since 2004 and exists solely on egg white omelets with spinach and muffins made with powdered milk, egg whites and stevia. She could feed a small country Hollandaise for months with all the yolks she tosses.) We watched bad TV and then we ate some more. Before I headed back to DC on Sunday, we paid a visit to my oldest friend, Michelle.

Michelle and I have been friends since we were five, and inseparable since we were nine. She is by far the funniest person I know and I don't think I have one memory from childhood that doesn't involve her. She was the shit-stirrer in high school, the one always causing some kind of trouble; in fact, her senior year high school quote was, "If you have nothing nice to say, come sit by me." She has always been the fearless one, the outspoken one, the only person I know that can drive on the Long Island Expressway at 80 mph with her knee while applying liquid eyeliner perfectly.

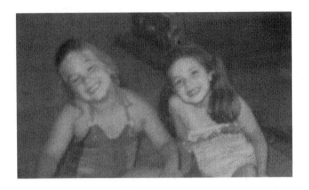

Me & Michelle, circa the 80's at Bar-H Day Camp

Our friendship was maintained long-distance when I came to Washington, DC in 1996 for college and she remained on Long Island. At 32, we were still as close as we were in high school, talking on the phone every other day, if not more. She was now married with a child and as I played with her son, Aiden, Michelle and I kind of looked at each other, got teary and then looked away, both of us unable to grasp what was actually happening and neither of us really wanted to talk about what was going to happen once I got back to DC, so we didn't. We hugged, told each other that we loved one another as we always do, and hours later, I was back on the train, headed back to DC and ready for the next phase.

That Wednesday was my biopsy. About two weeks prior I had resigned from my job as an account manager at a small marketing and communications firm trying to make HVAC units sound sexy and cool and Tuesday was my last day. My new job, making mixed used developments and apartment complexes sound sexy and cool wasn't slated to start until the following Monday, so the only calendar-bound thing standing in the way between me and my new job was this biopsy. As much as my mother begged and pleaded to come back to DC with me, I wasn't ready for her to join me on this proverbial bump in the road. This was nothing and I was fully prepared to do this alone. Ok, so you legally can't go to a biopsy yourself since you get lots of numbing medications that could impair your driving capabilities, so I bit the bullet and asked my best friend Pleasance to come with me. I try to avoid asking friends for favors, especially ones that involve them sitting in a waiting room for almost two hours on a Wednesday morning when they have kids and a life of their own.

So rather than spending my day basking in the three day vacation before starting my new job, I was repeatedly jabbed with a small needle to remove parts of this mystery dark cloud on my left breast. The doctor tried to make small talk, during which I tried to be totally causal since I was very sure that there was no way that I could have cancer. I told the doctor about the new job I was going to be starting that Monday, and how I had just finished grad school and recently ended a long-term relationship. I told him how happy and amazingly free I felt. Looking back, I can't believe how cavalier I was about the whole encounter, but I really was convinced that there wasn't anything wrong with me. Or perhaps I was in denial.

But either way, clearly, I was wrong (You're reading this book, after all). Two days later, I was having coffee with Pleasance in her kitchen, having just spent the night at her house because her husband was out of town. We were laughing about the previous night's events and playing with her then-two year old daughter Saylor who was eating breakfast with us. We were having a great time until I got a call from my gynecologist with the results of my biopsy.

"Are you at work?"

"No…why?"

"Are you alone?"

"No…why?"

"Because I have the results of your biopsy and I hate to tell you this, but you have cancer.

"Are you serious?"

I looked up at Pleasance and burst into tears. I remember that first look of hopelessness that came across her face. Pleasance had been my family since we met freshman year at George Washington University and I spent our first year of college sleeping in-between her and my other roommate Chrys on the floor of their double, when my bed sat, unused just five feet away in the larger room of our six person dorm room. The three of us were inseparable from day one, going through almost every type of drama together—marriage, babies, breakups, broken engagements and now, 15 years later, I stood in Pleasance's house, blindsided by cancer. This wasn't going to be something that could be fixed by having a talk or working it out. This was going to be harder than any other previous drama either of us had ever experienced. When we looked at one another, we both knew. As she watched me cry, her eyes filled with tears that she tried to swallow, not wanting to lose it completely in front of her daughter. One of the first things Pleasance said to me back in 1996 as I said goodbye to my parents while standing in the middle of my new home in room 728 of Thurston Hall was, "Please don't cry. If you cry, I'll cry." It's been that way ever since.

The next call was even harder to swallow, because I had to call my parents and tell them what was going on. After a good 15 minutes of trying to compose myself long enough to actually make the call, I finally hit send and my mom immediately answered.

"You aren't going to believe this" I said rather than hello.

"Meredith, what is it. Is it cancer?"

"I. HAVE. CANCER." I yelled into the phone and then immediately felt guilty for Saylor, Pleasance's daughter who just heard Auntie Mer scream, yell and cry all in the matter of an hour.

Despite my reluctance to have my parents drop whatever it was that they were doing and come down to DC, I didn't really have a choice. I didn't have the mental capacity to wrap my brain around the barrage of doctor's appointments, MRI's, PET scans and additional biopsies that I was about to be subjected to. Not only did I have to find a slew of new doctors, but I also had to push back the start date of my new job, which had me terrified. Intellectually, I was ready to be "on top of my shit," and the idea of pushing back the start date of a new job challenged my idea of what being a good new employee looked like. But I knew I needed to, despite my fear of making a bad first impression. The worst part was an even deeper fear: I had no idea if I'd even have a job after all this.

Legally, I didn't need to tell my new office what was going on. So I chose to stay in the cancer-closet for the time being, and simply stated that I had an emergency and would need to push my start date back one week. They agreed, thankfully and I had the week free to dive right into the cancer pool, which included some of the best and worst moments of my life where I was reminded of just how lucky I was to have two parents who would drop anything to help and a circle of friends who did whatever I asked of them, which was just to keep me laughing no matter what.

Chapter 2: Building Your Teams (August 2010 - September 2010)

After your diagnosis, the dust of the initial shock will settle, at which point, there will likely be a sense of overwhelming urgency that will take over your entire life. It's almost like the world is moving forward at double-speed, and yet there you are standing in the middle, watching it happen. You know you need to get up and move, but you just don't know the best direction in which to move first. There are doctors that need to be found, friends that need to be told the news, and essentially an entire army of support needs to be put into place. I like to call this "building your special teams." It's definitely overwhelming: I remember that I was simultaneously telling close friends and family about what was happening in between running to meet oncologists, plastic surgeons and general surgeons. I was exhausted, and you'll probably be exhausted too.

The other thing that will probably happen is that you'll get sick of yourself. What do I mean? Well, let me put it this way: you will find yourself talking about yourself for days and days to different people. By the end of my first week dealing with cancer, I was already sick of hearing my own voice and listening to my story. I was tired of telling every new doctor every detail of my life— I almost wished I had hired a spokesperson so I could just walk into an office, take my shirt off and have someone else do the work of self-summary for me. Every time I would have to talk to any doctor or friend, I tended to get all teary and anxious, having no idea what was going to happen next. If I could've avoided that from time to time, it might've been nice.

Building Your Emotional Team

This is the part of the journey where you will need—not just want—friends. I will tell you this bluntly: if you don't have any friends, I highly suggest you find some, fast. These people will not only make you laugh when you need to, cry when you need to, and be there when you want to Hulk out, but they will also shock you with regard to how much they care. You may not think you need that much care, but it goes a long way, I promise you.

I had a two-pronged approach when building my emotional team: I ended up with Team Friend and Team Family.

Team Friend

Some people are able to collect friends throughout their lives, like Garbage Pail Kids, and keep those connections for years and years. Others have one or two close confidantes that they turn to in times of need. And of course, there are those that trust virtually no one and choose only to maintain a smattering of loose connections— those people who are great for a drink after work or dinner on a weeknight…and that's about it.

In your 20s and 30s, you have all different friend circles. There are your college friends and your new work friends, and a very lucky few still have their high school friends. And to top it off, there are also usually those friends you just happen to pick up along the way— the friends of friends, the girlfriends of college boyfriends and variations thereof. The greatest thing about having lots of people come in and out of your life is that you get to develop friendships along the way as all of you grow and change. Some of the people that you may have come to depend on fade into the woodwork due lifestyle changes or moves, and some that had been peripheral friends may come into the foreground. I always found it so strange that some of my closest girlfriends in my 30s were people that I had gone to college with, meaning that we didn't even know each other until midway through our 20s. It's funny how relationships change.

My rule of thumb was always to let friendships evolve as they may, and of course, there were friends that I lost along the way. But most of them were still there, and this allowed me to turn to all of the people that I'd ever cried and laughed with once I was diagnosed.

Breaking the news to your friends that you have cancer can be daunting. It's a worse version of telling them that you've quit your job or broke up with a guy that everyone liked. One important factor to remember when breaking this news to your friends is that this is *your* deal— your fight not theirs. So if you have friends that you're worried about upsetting or angering, then think of it this way: those people probably shouldn't be in your inner circle anyway. Coming from someone who was always "the fixer," and often "the people-pleaser" I had to find it within myself to let those identities go when I came out with my diagnosis. Your body is a full time job, and to put it bluntly, you don't and won't have time to deal with the bullshit.

Set your terms with your friends. Let them know what you expect of them, what you'll need from them. If you don't want people calling you once a day just to make sure you're OK, Tell them. It's OK to not want that. If you've had problems asking for help in the past, now's the time to let your pals know that that might change: as independent as you think you are, you can't go through this process alone and without support.

I dealt with this every day, since I was (and will always try to be) the most independent woman there is. I can live alone, sure. But I used to find myself thinking constantly, "Oh I can go to this doctor's appointment by myself, no problem. I can go look at wigs on the off chance I lose all of my hair by myself." But here's the thing: no, you can't. You're going to need those friends around you to tell you that the pink wig that you're about to purchase does not make you look good, it makes you look like a moron. This was a concept that I had a lot of trouble grasping, especially in the beginning.

The hard part is figuring out how to let them know what's going on. If you're a pretty private person, like I was at the time, you don't want anyone to know anything is different, that anything is changing. You are still the same person, and as much as you don't want people to look at you differently just because you have cancer, they will. They'll try not to, but they will, and it's OK. You would do it, too. Shortly after my diagnosis I was invited to a raw food dinner featuring Kris Carr, the author of *Crazy Sexy Cancer* and was lucky enough to hear her tell her story. As I sat and sipped on my cold soup, wondering how anyone could eat raw food all of the time, I listened to Kris tell her story. She had received her diagnosis at around the same age that I did a few years before and she told the audience: "To my friends, I signified death. I made them look at death and the fact that we will all eventually die."

I almost choked on my kale crouton. Was that how everyone sees me? I didn't want that. Going through something like this in your 20s and 30s is a really hard pill to swallow. There's nothing about it that's fair or necessarily fun, but having a great group of people by your side is nothing short of a miracle drug. I love to laugh, I love to joke, I love people around me that make me laugh and to hear someone make a joke or send a funny text message was really what got me through some of the really bad days of treatment or days when I just felt defeated.

Laughing about a funny joke or movie with friends on a tough day was always healing—but the humor that was most important for me to cultivate was about the situation overall: I wanted everyone know that it was OK to laugh about all the craziness that was going on in my life. Of course, I took the lead on this, joking that I never wanted to wait in line because I had cancer or using my illness as an excuse not to do something. "What? You want me to go to this party?" I'd say "Nah, I have cancer, don't feel like it." It was most important to me for my friends and family know that it was OK to ask questions, that this wasn't a death sentence and that I was not curled in a ball in the corner of my apartment, waiting to die, because I knew from day one that becoming a cancer statistic just wasn't in the cards for me. There was no way I was going to die; I had too many one-liners that still needed to be delivered.

Your diagnosis, however promising it may be, will affect everyone around you. Your friends, your family, your coworkers, everyone will all look at you differently no matter how hard you try to maintain a sense of normalcy. For some, the onslaught of increased communication may be a welcome addition to daily life; for others, there is nothing worse than the thought of the same person calling you every single day to ask, "How are you feeling today?" The reality is that you'll have the same answer for at least a year, and that answer will be something along the lines of, "tired." Navigating these communication-waters can be tricky. While you know your friends' care is all coming from a wonderful place, there are going to be days where you want to hurl your phone across the room and hide under your bed. On those days, I strongly recommend not breaking any type of machinery because you'll just have to leave the house to get it fixed at some later date, leaving you open to interactions with even more annoying people.

Whatever the circumstances are around your illness, it's always hard to read how your friends are going to react so to give you some perspective on some of their possible reactions, I went right to the source. I asked my four closest and oldest friends: Michelle (my best friend since Kindergarten), Pleasance (my yoda, yin to my yang), Chrys (my roommate of seven years and, had we lived in another state, my life partner) and Rick (Chrys' husband and my undisputed twin) about how they felt about the situation and what feelings the news had evoked within them.

Michelle

"When you told me the news that no friend wants to tell, never once did the movie Beaches flash through my head, never once did I think to myself, 'Can I lose my BFF?' never once did I think I would be 'walking' for you on one day. NEVER.

Once you told me the news that you probably knew all along, I knew what was going on, but didn't really want to believe it. Everything happened rather quickly, in mind, that is. I spoke to Rich (my husband) and my parents but no matter how many times it was spoken about, I just still didn't get it. There is no book for this kind of crap. So I kind of did what I normally would do and made you laugh, talked to you for a while and made sure you were OK and were still speaking about what was going on without going into detail that you didn't want to get into.

To be honest, this entire ordeal really hit me after my first visit to DC after your major operation. My mind was going crazy on that short plane ride to DC. Was I going to open the door and see my best friend 'sick'? Would I be able to handle that? Why was I making this about me? Oh my god a million thoughts until I opened the door and was greeted by...you...just you...same ol' you. If I hadn't had a family of my own, I would have never left. I would have figured out a way to move Rich to DC and start our lives there because leaving that Sunday afternoon broke my heart. I have been visiting DC for years and never once did I cry like a baby when leaving. I am always sad to say bye to you but know that we will talk in an hour once I land...this time though...this time the cab driver had to ask if I was ok. I cried not because I thought you were going anywhere, because I knew you were beating this shit the entire time, but I cried because I felt helpless. How the fuck does a person get their best friend through something like cancer?"

Michelle's response is in no doubt similar to that of your best friend, if you are lucky enough to have someone in your life for as long as Michelle has been in mine. She was my first official visitor after my surgery, after my mother who had been living in my studio apartment with me for almost a month. By the time Michelle had arrived, I was ready for a new face. I was ready to get out of the house for more than a walk around the block, and I was ready to eat a meal somewhere other than on my couch. So off we went, me in my Victoria's Secret Pink sweatpants (since I was not yet able to wear real pants due to the incision running east-to-west below my belly button), and my medical-grade sports bra. Michelle kept clearing a path for me by elbowing people out of the way; "Move, dick," she would say to anyone who posed a threat to coming in contact with any part of my body. She was my own personal bodyguard, and I never wanted her to leave. When she did, my apartment was eerily quiet—particularly so because I was still healing from my surgery and wasn't working yet. I had days upon days with nothing to do. "I'll write that great American novel I've always wanted to finish," I thought to myself. "I'll go to every museum in Washington that I've always wanted to go to," I'd ponder. But these were lofty goals.

What I really did end up doing was spending a lot of time with Pleasance and Saylor. We ran errands, we went apple picking, we went to gymnastics class and I would get somewhat quizzical looks from the other mothers while I held Saylor's hand as she navigated the balance beam, probably wondering whether Pleasance and I were a couple, or if I was just the nanny.

During this time, I was pretty much in denial about having cancer and what it really meant, probably because I didn't really understand. And in fact, I don't think I *wanted* to understand. As I had expressed to my friends, I didn't want to be treated differently. "This is all a blip on my radar," I rationalized to them (and to myself), "Cancer will in no way define who I am."

But clearly, these words proved to be an impossibility as I learned that there's no way that cancer CAN'T change you. You will in no doubt come out on the other end a different person in one way or another no matter how hard you try not to. In the beginning, you will fight it with all of your might, and the whole thing will undoubtedly leave some friends baffled as to how to deal with you, even if you make it clear that you do not want to be "dealt with."

For Pleasance, my indifference and unwillingness to accept what was happening proved difficult for her as she is a "fixer". When an issue is presented, she wants to swoop in and help. So when I insisted that everything was fine, that nothing needed to be fixed, it frustrated her I think.

Pleasance and my relationship had been sisterly within the first hour we met. Both being only children meant that we both felt this inherent need to watch out for one another. To this day, we are completely intertwined in one another's lives and have been for a while now. This made her reaction to my diagnosis a lot more visceral, not to mention the fact that shortly after I had been diagnosed, Pleasance learned that she was pregnant with her second child.

Pleasance

"I really, really didn't think it would end up being cancer. I was so sure that it was just a scare and we'd get through it like everything else and life would go on as usual.

The night before we found out it was truly cancer, we had been out having a blast. Feeling good, and just being. This was the last cancer-free night. I remember so very clearly going to bed that night. My husband was away and Meredith was staying with me. We woke up cozy, comfy and calm, a lightness I don't think we'll ever have again, an immaturity that was soon to fade as soon as the call came in. Plans needed to be made, doctors, appointments, health insurance and holding on the phone for what seemed like forever. I went numb and I went into mom mode. I wanted to take care of her. I did not want her at any appointment alone, I had a million questions. What was going to happen? What were the next steps? What did we need to do?

I became obsessed with cancer in young adult—searching them out, emailing them and asking more questions. I called Meredith numerous times a day. I remained very involved, very protective of her and made sure to stay on top of what was happening.

Soon after, I found out I was pregnant with my second child. I felt horrible; how could I have a life growing inside of me while I was so desperately trying to "save" my best friend? How could I have joy when she had so many struggles? I felt physically sick and depressed about the pregnancy occurring at the same time as the cancer. I wasn't sure I would be able to deal with both. I had friends and family tell me to back off, and that I was getting too involved. For me, there's no way I could ever be too involved in Meredith's life. We are still only children and have vowed to be each other's sisters. She is the closest thing I have to a sister, closer probably than a "real" sister. I would get very annoyed and irritated when people would tell me to take space because Meredith and I don't take space on anything.

To be perfectly honest, I didn't think about her length of life. Everyone said she was going to be fine but I wasn't sure what to believe given all I had read and the fact that I thought there was no way she could have cancer to begin with, how could I know if she'd survive? I struggled deeply with another huge issue for our family. Meredith is our daughter's guardian if something happens to my husband and I. What now? Do you make her the guardian of the new baby too knowing about the cancer?

These were huge questions, big choices I was not ready to make, topics I didn't want to think about. I felt SELFISH and scared. I'm a realist and the realities were freaking me out. I disconnected from friends and family and just poured myself into the healing, nurturing and care taking of my unborn baby and my best friend.

We spent many afternoons just sitting in her apartment. Me sleeping, Meredith entertaining my daughter, just watching TV and doing nothing; it felt a lot like college as the days passed by. Over time, we began to notice the very strong similarities between pregnancy and cancer, especially as Meredith was going through chemotherapy. Exhaustion, nausea, aversion to foods, good days and bad days, fear, overwhelmed but with one big difference at the end of my year I would have a son. And at the end of hers, she would HOPEFULLY be cancer free. The guilt was palpable."

I am a lucky girl in more ways that I care to count. I don't know what I did in life to deserve to find a roommate like Chrys, but the George Washington University housing gods were smiling on me the day they placed me in a room with Pleasance and Chrys.

Chrys is the only roommate I've ever had post-college, and she set the bar pretty high for my boyfriend as I am sure that he will never be a better roommate than Chrys. Though I should note that we affectionately call her Babby now, due to her former New Jersey accent and corresponding Jersey nails (that have since been filed down to normal human length), which made her remind an old college friend of Barbara Streisand. The nickname originated in 2000 and has stuck so well that now even Chrys' husband Ricky will call her Babby. Chrys cleans, she cooks, she will watch endless amount of bad TV with me without judging how long we've been sitting there doing virtually nothing. Not only is she the type of friend who will pick me up and take me wherever I need to go, since she has a car and I don't, but on the ride, she will give the best television recaps of any TV show. She is not only my human DVR, she is also my sounding board, my confidant and a friend that has never nor will judge me and my antics.

In our seven years of living together, and an upwards of 15 years of being friends, we've only been in one major fight that I can remember in 2003 and rather than let her drive away angry, I opened her car door, hopped into the driver's seat and wouldn't let her leave until she was no long upset with me. Sometimes, we sit on the phone and watch TV together because it reminds us of when we lived together and were just starting to figure out what being an adult really meant. I think because we went through that formative post-college time together, she knows my moods and mannerisms better than anyone.

Chrys

"How could she possibly have cancer? She is too young. This is a mistake. It will be minor. The tests will come out clean. It's going to be benign.

It's not benign, but it will be small and isolated. It had spread more than we thought. She won't need chemo, radiation at the most.

She needs both chemo and radiation. How the hell did this happen?

As the bad news kept pouring in, there was one very significant small miracle that always stayed in the front of my thoughts—how were we lucky enough to find out from a stupid pulled muscle in her chest that she had an advanced stage of breast cancer?

The day we found out it was cancer was the scariest day of my life. Is my best friend going to beat this? Is she going to lose her hair? Is she going to be in pain all the time? It was the day that started my own cycle of random crying outbursts as I watched her go through the shittiest year possible, after what I thought was the shittiest year prior with regards to her relationship with her ex-fiancé. I cried when I was by myself just thinking about it, but that was my own private experience. I never cried with her...Well just once, when she first found out and we were sitting in her apartment, but that ended in laughter as all of our conversations do. And I'm glad we had that moment because it was then that I realized that cancer may be the reality but when we were together, it will not get the serious undercurrent it carries. I made the decision to just keep laughing with her through this, like always, because it's what makes her happy. It's why our relationship is always so easy and enjoyable. SCREW YOU CANCER, we laugh at you. You are not going to scare us and you most certainly are not going to change us.

The whole situation was a miracle of circumstances, things happening at the right time to avert what could have been a worse situation. That stupid pulled muscle saved her damn life, and consequently mine because she is still here. I still get to talk to her ten times a day, and we will continue to make jokes, laugh all the time, and she will continue to be my best friend. Cancer – 0, us – 1. But please, Universe, no rematch."

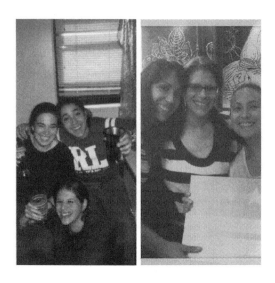

Selma, Patty & Mer. L. 1996, R. 2014

I've often heard that women marry men who are like their fathers, but in Chrys' case, she married a man who is just like me so naturally, I'm kind of obsessed with him. Chrys and Ricky met our first year out of college when we each had our first real grown-up jobs. I was a matchmaker for a dating service (before the advent of online dating) and Chrys was a civics tour guide of Washington, DC for a company that would bring in students from all over the US to DC for a week and she would teach them about politics and show them around.

After her first day, we convened on our Golden Girl's inspired pink floral and wicker couch to talk about her day.

"I made two new friends from Ohio. Their names are Ricky and Adam and they're nice. We're going to meet them for drinks tomorrow."

"Cool," I said.

My first conversation with Ricky went like this:

"I make the best Bundt cake," he said.

"Oh really?" I asked, already thinking that this kid was beyond bizarre.

"Want to see the recipe?" he asked as he pulled it out of his wallet. It was folded in fours on a pastel post-it and had clearly been in there for a while.

"Umm, sure."

On our way home, I expressed my concern to Chrys that while Adam seemed perfectly normal and nice, Ricky was a loose cannon.

"That kid is weird."

Fast forward a month, at which point Ricky had become a permanent fixture on our couch, making it painfully obvious that he was in love with Chrys, even though they were just friends. But Ricky used every excuse he could to be around all of the time. If Chrys wasn't home, he'd wait for her and since I was home a lot more than she was, Ricky and I spent a lot of time together. A lot. So much so that after a while, we just started going out together to pass the time until Chrys came home from dates with older men that Ricky and I would mercilessly make fun of. Eventually, Chrys gave in and they started dating. Eight years later, they got married.

Ricky quickly became the brother I never thought I wanted but loved having around. We tag-team making fun of Chrys, we were the last ones out until last call and we both talk non-stop about our love of food. There was a time before Chrys and Ricky moved in together where the three of us lived together in a *Three's Company*-esque situation. Just like in the sitcom, a strange man once emerged from my room while Ricky was getting ready for work. They nodded at one another and as I made my way towards the shower, Ricky stood in the kitchen, shaking his head at me. I'm also convinced that when I was away on a business trip, he ate my goldfish in retaliation for me always eating the ice cream he kept in the freezer even though I have been lactose intolerant since I was a teenager.

Now fast forward to today, where Ricky and I gossip like two old women over text message about anyone and everyone and he will always have an opinion about everything I do. I'm OK with that, because like any male/female relationship, I have learned to tune him out and vice versa.

Having your girlfriends respond to breast cancer, or any cancer, is different from dealing with your male friends since there can be a closeness with your female friends that some people don't necessarily have with their male friends. This wasn't the case with Ricky since at the time of diagnosis, we were as close as many of my girlfriends.

Ricky

"Meredith and I are very similar in more ways than one can possibly imagine, which means she is a great 'second wife' and an even better friend. One of our defining characteristics is that we would both

much rather ignore, avoid and/or deny tough situations at all costs ... and up until that day this method had worked pretty well.

When she was diagnosed, I cycled through the spectrum of emotions—shock, pain, sadness, shit, what the fuck, why, how—but my prevailing thought was why couldn't this happen to me instead? I couldn't stand to see my friend hurt, confused, living by herself and muddling through a battle with a life-threatening disease. Call it the protective little brother in me, call it human nature, but Meredith didn't deserve this and I would've much rather carried this burden for her.

Once I processed everything, I knew this was real and that I wouldn't be able to transfer the cancer to myself. So I did the next best thing: I called my childhood best friend, an oncologist who Meredith knows and loves, and this turned out to be the most helpful thing I could do for her. He could talk to her in a way that none of us could. As a doctor, he could help her understand what she was about to go through, and arm her with knowledge and all the right questions to ask—but most importantly, he could do this in a warm, non-doctor sort of way.

I decided that I would do what I always do: ignore the problem. I continued to text Meredith, joke with her, make fun of her and do all the things we always did, but it just happened to be while she was being pumped full of drugs with an arctic cap on her head, or laying on the couch recovering from chemotherapy. This was my way of helping—assuring her that things would be OK and continue to be as normal as possible. I knew that once I started addressing the elephant in the room, she would know it was time to panic.

When all was said and done, I realized that things happen for a reason. At least for the time being, the best thing possible for Meredith and all our friends was that she got cancer and not me. Why? Because apparently all those hangovers Meredith has pulled herself up from over the past decade prepared her for the hell she experienced. I promise you this: if I had cancer, I would be the annoying, needy and complaining friend to the point where people would wish they had cancer just to shut me up. Fortunately, now all is right with the world and I can go back to pretending none of this happened. Anyone in the mood for some Bundt cake?

If it weren't for my group of friends, I would not have been able to make it through my diagnosis, treatment and everything else that came after. They helped me with everything from keeping my spirits up when I couldn't find a job, to laughing with me as I navigated the online dating scene post-treatment, and everything else along the way.

But now, let me tell you a bit about Team Family…

Team Family

Living in DC and having my parents in New York has meant that my friends usually function as my immediate family members. But dealing with your actual family can be a whole other animal in all facets of life, depending on your family dynamic. As an only child, I didn't really have a choice in the level of involvement that my parents had in my treatment; understandably, I have always been their main focus and looking back on it now, I know that I would not have been able to handle my illness without them (even when they were stepping out in the middle of my chemo treatments to smoke and garnering looks of disapproval from my fellow patients).

Growing up as an only child is a double-edged sword. While you get more of the advantages that you probably wouldn't have had if there were a fourth person in the family (a dog, summers at sleep-away camp and an overpriced secondary and graduate education), you're also in the full spotlight of your parents' attention all the time. They will be highly attentive to your grades, your friends, where you're going, who you're going out with. And let me tell you, it can be a lot to handle.

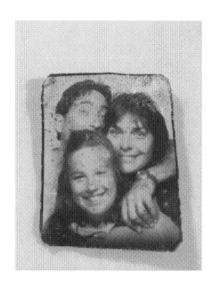

The day before my first summer at sleepaway camp, circa 1988ish.

As I got older, I tried my best to distance myself from my parents, which was one of the main reasons that my post-college plans included remaining in DC rather than returning to New York. There was a nice sense of balance to that distance—being a 30-minute plane ride away from my parents so that I was close to them, but could still cultivate my own life. My mother and I have a very typical mother-daughter relationship: she pries and I get annoyed, but I call her every day because if I don't, something just feels off. We definitely had our extremely tumultuous phase for most of my teenage years, with fights so vicious that one or two of them ended in physical altercations. I attribute these particularly intense fights to my mom's constant fear that I was going to leave and never return, which is another downside to being an only child—there's no one else to worry about. When I would go out at night in high school, I'd leave notes of what I was wearing so on the off chance I never made it home, she'd know what to tell the police. Once I left for college, our relationship changed for the better. Now with some space away from one another, my mother no longer feared that I would disappear into the night.

My relationship with my father is atypical, or at least I feel like it always was. But some of my best memories of my childhood involve him. We would make up songs and play the guitar and write stories together, as I hovered over him in his office as he clicked away on his typewriter, an artifact that he still uses. You can always hear when he's working in his office; there will be the continual click, click, click, ding of the typewriter. I think he's the only person that still actively looks for whiteout.

To watch a father deal with his daughter's breast cancer is no doubt different for every father/daughter duo. I couldn't look my father in the eye at doctor's appointments or when we were even talking about what was happening because I would uncontrollably burst into tears and to this day, I cannot explain why. My father was never the dad that wanted a son and would make me do son-like things like mow the lawn or play football in the yard. He was more of a "let's listen to this Dave Brubeck album and I'll teach you about using the brush on a drum." Our family dinners, when we had them almost always involved the record player. We'd each get a turn picking out what we wanted to listen to. Mine was ALWAYS Barry Manilow, because I was convinced that Mandy was about my next door neighbor Amanda. My mom always chose either The Beatles or The Rolling Stones and my father tended toward classical—Bach, Beethoven, Brams. These are all what I grew up listening to during meals.

    Music always played a large part in my childhood, whether it was our dinner playlists or as a form of punishment. When I was 6 years old, the repercussion of drawing on my bedroom wall was to watch MTV all day and hit "record" on the VCR whenever a Bruce Springsteen video came on for my mother's own personal collection. As I grew up, I associated all types of music with my parents, each genre evoking a different emotion and in some ways, this still holds true today. I can't hear Bruce without thinking of my mother and any classical music piece sounds familiar to me and reminds me of sitting at the dining room table, my father at the head, my mother sitting across from me, chicken, in one form or another on our plates, and music filling the room.

My father never seemed to get involved in the mess that was my teenage years, other than being my SAT tutor, which was a mistake of gargantuan proportions. While most kids were being shuttled off to Kaplan, there I sat at my dining room table, flinging calculators across the room out of frustration. I was never good at math and my father always said it's because I was afraid of it, which was never the case. I cannot add—it's a known fact amongst my friends, comical at this point, but not so much when I was 16 years old.

Our relationship didn't change that drastically when I moved away. I would come home during college break and he would ask what I was reading, as we had both been English Lit majors during undergrad. I'd tell him and he'd shake his head in disapproval.

"What are they teaching you at that school? What am I paying for?" His tuition check was finally vindicated when I spent one month on *Finnegan's Wake*, one of my father's favorites, although he believed that I should have taken an entire semester on Joyce like he did back in the 60's.

My parents never played a big part in my decision making once I was out of college and living on my own until I turned 30 and found myself engaged to someone that they didn't necessarily love, or like for that matter. They had met my then-fiancée once or twice and while my father, who had never even spoken to me about dating or sex (he claims that when I was a few months old he told me all about the birds and the bees and concluded the conversation with "and don't ask me again") he actually had an opinion about this next step.

So, there I was, at 30 with my boyfriend of almost two years, down on one knee at a restaurant, totally blindsided. "This is what I've always wanted, isn't it?" I thought to myself as I saw him slowly sliding onto the floor with a small navy blue box. "This is what I'm supposed to be doing," I convinced myself as the word "Yes" slipped out of my mouth.

"Do my parents know," I asked?

I learned that my boyfriend had called them a number of times and they had not called him back. I never realized, until at least a year after the dust had settled they hadn't called him back with reason. They weren't behind me for the first time in my life. They didn't agree with a major life decision.

"Are you sure this is what you want?" my father asked me a few weeks into my engagement.

"Yes," I replied, although that wasn't necessarily true and I knew it wasn't because I couldn't look my father in the eye without crying.

For many fathers and daughters there's a "whatever my little girl wants" theme that runs throughout their life. And this is often especially the case with only children. My father and I weren't like that until I got sick. Even then, I wasn't asking for much. It was more out of sheer panic that I would turn to my father for help.

Emotionally, some people may find it difficult to reach out to their parents during this time since with younger cases of cancer, your parents will take the blame for your illness, even though, it's more than likely not their fault. Only 5% to 10% of breast cancers are thought to be hereditary, caused by abnormal genes passed from parent to child.[3] My parents couldn't help that they were both from Ashkenazi families, which also is a factor with all cancers. (The Jews could never catch a break.)

In my case, my breast cancer was not hereditary. My BRCA (Breast Cancer Susceptibility Gene) test had come back negative, meaning that there's no way my mother or my father could have passed the breast cancer gene along to me, a notion that we were all relieved to find out. The human genes known as BRCA1 and BRCA2 belong to a class of genes known as tumor suppressors. Mutation of these genes has been linked to hereditary breast and ovarian cancer.

Unsurprisingly, a woman's risk of developing breast and/or ovarian cancer is greatly increased if she inherits the BRCA1 or BRCA2 mutation. And believe it or not, men with these mutations also have an increased risk of breast cancer. Both men and women who have harmful BRCA1 or BRCA2 mutations may also be at increased risk of other cancers, not just breast cancer.[4]

Genetically-speaking, my parents were not the cause of my breast cancer. I never asked my father outright if he felt responsible for what was going on in any way, but my mother made it very clear that she took full responsibility for my illness. This feeling threw her into a Jew-shame-spiral, which she made sure to bring up any chance she could. Here's an example of a daily phone call that we would have in between my treatments when they were in NY and I was resting in DC:

"How do you feel today," my mother would ask.
"I'm OK. Tired, my stomach is definitely off from the chemo."
"Ucch, my stomach is such a mess from all of this. I can't even eat I'm so upset."
"OK mom, I gotta go."

And that was the conversation.

My father would get on the phone and say:

"How are you feeling? Do you need money?"

And this was the way he dealt with it, the only way he really could—making sure that I was financially secure and had enough money on me at all times for every doctor's appointment, every medicine, anything I needed, which I will always be eternally grateful for since I was half working throughout my treatment and then subsequently found myself unemployed during the worst economic recession since the Great Depression.

The adage is, "You can choose your friends but you cannot choose your family," and there is never a time where this resonates more than when in the midst of a health crisis like cancer. But once you've stepped out of the cancer closet and have your support firmly in place, you can attack the next step: building your medical team. These are the people that are going to rebuild you and restore you to your former glory.

Building Your Medical Team

Understanding health care is like staring at one of those 3D pieces of artwork that were really popular in the 90's; you can gaze into the same piece of paper for hours and it just doesn't make sense. As much as I can tell you that you can let other people handle this for you, you can't. Cancer will become your full time job, regardless of what cancer you are diagnosed with. You will have more appointments with doctors that you never imagined possible. You will see a surgeon in the morning and an oncologist in the afternoon. Your plastic surgeon will be uptown and your therapist will be downtown. You will run all over the place and you will be exhausted. A small tip here, always have a book, a magazine or make sure your iPhone/iPad/iWhatever is charged the night before and you have a Mophie laying around. You will spend more time in waiting rooms surrounded by sicker people than you at times, and it's not fun. Bring your own entertainment.

    These doctors will become part of your life, you will collect them like baseball cards and it's almost a better way of looking at it; once you find out that you have cancer, you need to assemble a team that can bring home the championship.

    Everyone looks at finding physicians differently and I'm not going to sit here and tell you that men are better than women, or progressive doctors are better than traditional ones. Everything comes down to *your* comfort level. If you want only to work with women, then find women doctors. If you want only men, then find male doctors. After all, these people will see you at your most vulnerable.

In my case, I was topless more times than you care to count. I remember one moment at the end of my first week of non-stop doctor's appointments. After the 1,000th time taking off my shirt, I said, "At least during Mardi Gras, I got beads for this." Having breast cancer is like a long walk down Bourbon Street on Fat Tuesday, minus the hurricanes and the beads. More random people will see, touch, and inspect your body during breast cancer treatment than in college. Get used to it. It's for your own good.

There are a few key doctors that you will need and at any time of the week you will need to see them. The good news is you have cancer and not some random disease that you saw on an episode of *House*. Cancer is everywhere and there are thousands of doctors who are insanely well-equipped to treat you. The bad news is, well, you have cancer and as much as you don't want to deal with it, you have to.

The "Down There" People

If you are in your 20s and 30s and are a sexually active female, then your best friend is your gynecologist. If any of you think differently, then you're lying. I've been going to the same gynecologist since I was 20, and my file is about as long as this book. I call her for every itch, twinge, and inkling that something might be wrong and usually, up until this last visit, I was wrong. My doctor knows me so well, she actually called me after my surgery in the hospital to tell me that she had wanted to come by but had too many patients but wanted to check and see how I was doing.

Barring any sexual mishaps or pregnancy scares, which I'm sure we've all had, you see your gynecologist once a year for your general look under the hood and complimentary boob squeeze. Most studies have recommended that women with no family history of breast cancer start getting yearly mammography's at 35, until then it's typically done manually by your gynecologist.

We all know that we're supposed to check ourselves regularly just like Brenda and Kelly did on *Beverly Hills 90210* when Brenda missed her SAT's because of her breast cancer scare, but I know very few women who actually do it, especially in my age bracket. I wasn't even looking when I found mine; I had just kind of rolled over onto it and thought, "Hmm, that feels weird. Oh well, time for bed." But just in case you were wondering, that's not what you're supposed to do. If you ever feel anything, run (don't walk) to your gynecologist since early detection is all the rage these days.

According to contemporary research, mammography is one of the most effective modalities for prevention. According to Cancer.org's most recent report, "Mammography can often detect breast cancer at an early stage, when treatment is more effective and a cure is more likely. Numerous studies have shown that early detection saves lives and increases treatment options." Moreover, the report shows that since 1990, there have been steady declines in breast cancer mortality among women. The reason? "…a combination of early detection and improvements in treatment." In women without symptoms, mammography still reportedly is able to detect 80 – 90% of breast cancer. [5]

When I finally made the appointment to get my breast checked, it was the gynecologist that I went to first. You want to make sure that you have an office you trust with a doctor who you like, and it's always good to ask your friends for a recommendation if you need one. In fact, have at least five friends that go to the same office I do, which is always fun to run into a friend in the waiting room. A good gynecologist is like having that perfect black dress, comforting and reliable.

If you don't have a good gynecologist or one that you particularly like, do some research. Asking your friends can be a great place to start, but so is the Internet. This is one of the only appropriate forms of Googling that won't throw you into a tailspin. When it comes to researching medical issues, the Internet usually functions as an intricate plan to freak the shit out of people all over the world with stories of spontaneous combustion and fallen limbs. So, do yourself a favor and please try to stay away from these stories. For most women, going to the gynecologist is about as fun as having a rabid beast gnaw on your arm in the first place. You don't need to read about a woman who went in to the gynecologist for her annual and came out with a baby. These stories DO exist, but if you're reading this book, you already know that that probably isn't in the cards for you. The best source for finding a doctor that you have any chance of liking besides asking your friends is consulting with your primary health care provider.

Please allow at least 30 minutes for this call or Internet search. With the onslaught of social media today, we depend on our peers to do the guinea-pigging for us, not the other way around. You'd be surprised about how many doctors and other professionals have a strong social media presence, it's unreal. But it's your job to weed out the crap and find a practice that you are going to like, one that is convenient for you and one that you feel you want to grow with. It's kind of like dating, actually. Put the time in, do your research and don't give up because the right one IS out there!

And so concludes my "You can do it!" speech about finding a gynecologist.

The Antiseptic Surgeon

Once you have been diagnosed, information will be thrown at you at an alarming rate, like a rapid fire of instructions from doctors, family members, friends, and even random strangers you'll meet in waiting rooms. This is where trusting your gynecologist comes in handy, or at least it did in my case. Once my biopsy had come back positive, I was faced with a number of appointments that had to be made rather quickly. Because of the size of my tumor, .8 cm, which is relatively small, and since the cancer had not spread elsewhere, I was looking at a lumpectomy.

But who would perform such a task? This is where you find a surgeon, or more specifically, a general surgeon who, ideally specializes in breast diseases and also has experience with lymph node surgeries (either sentinel or bilateral). As I said, my surgeon was recommended to me by my gynecologist's office and what I soon learned, at least in my experience is that many of these doctors all work together and recommend one another. Each time I went to a doctor and recited my ever-growing list of doctors I was working with, someone would say "Oh Ari" or "Oh Mike's great". I had no idea who these people were in the beginning and in reality I didn't care if I ever saw these people ever again.

Your surgeon is essentially your own personal hazmat team. He will take out the cancerous tumors and if needed, perform a lymph node biopsy. This is the procedure in which the surgeon takes a certain number of nodes out of your lymphatic system to test for positive nodes. A positive result means that the cancer has spread into the lymph system, which isn't a death sentence, but does mean that your course of treatment might be a little more than you had bargained for.

It's my own theory that you need to have a good rapport with all your doctors, especially your surgeon. Sure, I know that surgeons don't tend to be like annoyed waiters or waitresses who spit in your food; in the case that a surgeon doesn't like you, it's not as if they are going to botch your surgery on purpose. But I do think it's always easier if you are able to carry on a conversation with ANY doctor without feeling like you're being annoying. It's always good to remember that when you're visiting a doctor for the first time.

Essentially, you're interviewing them, and they'll be working for you, so don't feel like you're being a pest.

My surgeon Dr. P looks like a cross between Dick Butkus and Mike Ditka. I remember that he took the time to explain to me what a lumpectomy was and what it would entail, since this was my original course of treatment after we received the results of my first biopsy. It's a lot to swallow, but luckily when you are diagnosed with any form of cancer, you pretty much can become a walking pharmacy, should you choose. I had asked Dr. P if there was anything he could give me since I was having trouble sleeping since my diagnosis and his response was, "You're 32 and have just been diagnosed with breast cancer, you can have whatever you want." I walked out with a script for Ambien, Xanax and Valium (I only used the Xanax for fear of waking up in the middle of the night in an Ambien-induced binge fest), and an order for an MRI to make sure there weren't any other pesky tumors lurking around before they cut me open for a lumpectomy.

The MRI was a game-changer for me, for just past the .8 cm tumor that was found during my first mammogram lived a smaller .3

cm tumor that had not been detected. It's pretty amazing how technology is always trying to one-up itself, but it does, and there I was BACK on the table for image-guided core needle biopsy, round two. You keeping score? So far in two week period I had one sonogram, one mammogram, one MRI, and two biopsies.

    Due to the location of the smaller tumor, which was precariously close to the first one, Dr. P had no choice but to opt for a mastectomy on the left side rather than a lumpectomy as originally planned. The reasoning for this was as follows: in order to get both tumors, partial removal would be very invasive, and there would be too much disfiguration as a result. Plus, why would I take the chance to allow for the possibility of smaller tumors starting to grow in the same spot? Well, I wouldn't, which is why I listened to Dr. P. But it wasn't easy. The thought of having your breast operated at the age of 32 is hard enough, but to learn that they are going to be taking the ENTIRE left side was a whole other beast. There wasn't enough Xanax in the world to make this sound in any means OK with me, until I met my plastic surgeon and I learned about the only upside to breast cancer, a breast upgrade.

Plastics

As I said, everyone has their own criteria for choosing their doctor. When I emerged from the shock that I was losing a breast I had little knowledge of what this entailed or what happened next. Sure, I had seen images of women who had gone through mastectomies and had opted against reconstruction; this was not an option to me. I was 32 years old and recently single. There was no way that I was going to be OK with having a surgery that didn't leave me looking as close to the way I had always looked. Reconstruction was a must. I started doing my research.

My search began with the plastic surgeon that was recommended to my mother though my breast surgeon, but that wasn't good enough for me. I needed to know more. I needed to know where they were located. For me, location was key. If I'm going to a plastic surgeon, they need to be located in a place that typically sees a lot of women requesting "upkeep". For Washington, DC, this is typically in places like Fairfax, Virginia and Montgomery County, Maryland and in the district. These areas are known for women with lots of money and lots of fake boobs. I researched these doctors first.

In my cross referencing, I found that the surgeon that had been recommended to me fell into many of my criteria.

1. He was located in Chevy Chase, Maryland- a hot bed of plastic surgery activity.
2. He was young and attractive.
3. His office was located across the street from Jimmy Choo and Barney's, which is where all fancy women go after they have a chemical peel.
4. He had a great tie on in every piece of Googled material
5. He performed a surgery called a TRAM flap which essentially means that they take the fat from your stomach and put it in your breast to create a new breast that is natural.

Here was my reasoning with the TRAM flap rather than an implant. Since it was only my left side that was going to be removed, I feared that I would look uneven, like half Barbie doll, half human. This surgery allowed me to maintain a natural feel to my breast and as a bonus, a tummy tuck. I like to call this a win-win. Not too shabby, huh? I was willing to forgo the rock hard six-pack abs that I was never really destined to have in favor of a new breast that felt pretty similar to the original.

I never thought that I would be sitting in a waiting room to see a plastic surgeon, but sure enough, there I was, just weeks after my diagnosis in late August with my "cancer notebook" filled with questions for Dr. B, my new plastic surgeon. My cancer notebook was, in reality, a notebook where I kept every doctor's business card and various prescriptions for various pills that I had been given thus far.

Sitting in the plastic surgeon's office is kind of a weird experience; at least it was for me. As women came in and out, I wondered what about them was fake or stretched or pulled or pealed, not realizing that within a few weeks, I would be that woman and that people would be wondering the same thing about me. When you're faced with a surgery like a bilateral mastectomy, there's really nothing fun about it, so when the notion of getting to re-create a part of my body was the focus, I welcomed this event as almost comic relief.

A few days before my first appointment, Chrys and I were scouring the plastic surgeon's website for any inclination of what I was about to be subjected to.

"Oh, he's cute," Chrys said after clicking on the plastic surgeon's web bio.

There he was, the man who was going to rebuild me like Frankenstein, decked out in a white lab coat with a Burberry tie sticking out.

"What is he like 30?" I asked. "He looks rather young, don't you think?"

"I think he's hot. Let me come with you so I can meet him," Chrys joked. I was still insistent on going to all of my appointments alone.

"How about this? I'll scout the scene for you and then you can come to the next one."

For some reason, I had to have a plastic surgeon who matched my sardonic sense of humor, and I was lucky enough to have found him on my first try. After our initial meeting, and the ceremonial taking off of my shirt for the 100th time that week, we discussed options and right off the bat I said, "I don't want them to be fake," which I quickly learned is something that you don't really want to say to a plastic surgeon. It's kind of like telling a Top Chef that his food tastes just like Chef Boyardee.

Visiting your new plastic surgeon for the first time is an experience that you definitely want to be prepared for. I found that knowing my options in advance made our meeting a lot more productive. Rather than spending time going over the ins and outs of plastic surgery, which I had previously known nothing about other than what I had seen on *Nip/Tuck*, I was sure of my choices and what I wanted the end result to be. As scary as it looks, check out your plastic surgeon's website, read his or her bio, check out what kind of surgeries they do. That way, when the date of your appointment rolls around, you won't have a deer in headlights look when they're explaining what's going to happen. And try your best to pay attention during these conversations.

True story: I was maxed out on information and missed the part where my plastic surgeon told me that I wouldn't have a nipple on my left side post-surgery and would not be getting it back until after all of my treatments were complete. Imagine my surprise after my first visit back to the plastic surgeon about a week after I had gotten out of the hospital.

One of the attributes that I enjoyed most about my plastic surgeon (and still do) is his understanding of my position. I wasn't there because I wanted to be, I was there because I HAD to be and the end result of my breast reconstruction wasn't just going to be something that my husband would see, because I didn't have one. As someone who was single and dating, the end result, to me, had to be something I felt comfortable and confident about. I was willing to do whatever it took in order to accomplish that, even if it meant waiting over a year to have my surgery 100% complete.

Here's a perfect example of my relationship with my plastic surgeon. About a year after we first met, we celebrated our anniversary of working with one another with a high-five. If that's not love, then I don't know what is.

The All- Knowing Oncologist

Finding the right oncologist can be a daunting task. If you decide that you want to be forward thinking and involve yourself in any and every clinical trial, you might want to find a more progressive oncologist. If you want to do things by the book, then perhaps a more traditional oncologist will be more your speed. Of course, if you have no clue about anything along those lines, like I did, you really just want to find a doctor that you trust and doesn't make you feel any worse than you already do, emotionally speaking.

Once again, I had a vague sense of criteria for oncologists, especially since I knew I was going to be visiting them more often than not. After my second MRI and positive biopsy, it was pretty much written in stone that I would need to go through some form of chemotherapy, and therefore that I would be spending a lot of time with whomever I chose. My first lead came once again through my gynecologist and from there I started my Google due diligence. Another research tool I used from DC's lifestyle magazine, *The Washingtonian's* annual Top Doctor Issue where they listed most of the doctors in the city.

Another important criteria for me, was someone that was close to home. One of the luxuries of living in downtown DC is that many of the specialists are located in the middle of the city, which is where I happened to have been living at the time. Having no idea what the upcoming year was going to entail, I wanted to make sure I wasn't shuffling on the Metro every other day when I wasn't sure I was actually going to have the energy to do so.

When I had finally chosen a practice that was close to my home, my initial appointment had been made with the partner in the practice that was a bit older. I don't know why but something made me change my mind and I decided on a whim to cancel the appointment, and asked to see the other doctor. In all likelihood, this probably changed the entire course of my cancer and chemotherapy journey down the road.

Your first meeting with your oncologist will be frightening, or at least mine was. Once again, I opted to go alone, which, once again, was probably not the best decision. Armed only with my trusty cancer notebook, a Xanax and a pen, I walked into Dr. F's office for the first time. We looked each other up and down for a minute like we were both about to draw guns at 20 paces and then began our first conversation.

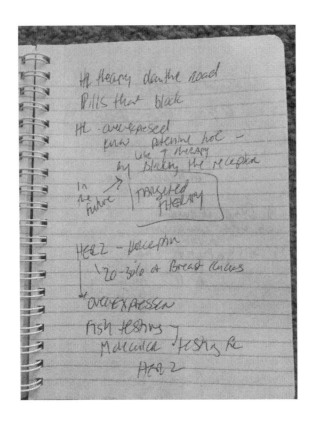

Notes from my first oncology appointment. Lots of arrows.

"So, tell me your story," he said, pen in hand, ready to transcribe.

I began my story from the very beginning, from the nasty encounter with the radiologist to the first biopsy, the scheduled lumpectomy the game changing MRI and then the second biopsy. He stopped me periodically to compare my story to the file that had already been compiled with my results. For a first meeting at a new office, I already had a file about 2 inches thick—pretty impressive. I like to call my oncologist "Ari the Onco" because it makes him sound funnier than he really is and we can all use as much humor as possible.

After speaking with Ari the Onco for about 40 minutes or so, he stopped and said "OK. You've had enough for one day. Come back in a few weeks after you've had some more time to heal and we'll talk more about your course of treatment." This made so much sense to me, why hadn't anyone done this with me before? By cutting short the conversation and saving more intricate talks for another time, I was not only able to digest what we had discussed but even more importantly, I was able to retain it. "I like you." I said, as I packed up and slowly eased myself out of the guest chair in his office. We shook hands and the rest is history. Ari the Onco and I will always continue to have a relationship and, barring a few bumps in the road, we've gotten along just fine.

The Therapist

I am a firm believer in therapy. As I'm not a big "group" person, I've always preferred one-on-one sessions. I think that having an already established relationship with a therapist really worked to my benefit once I was diagnosed because Dr. G, my therapist, already knew me pretty well.

Dr. G came into my life when I was at my lowest point. Ending an engagement is never fun, nor easy, especially when you aren't really sure what you want. I was pretty sure I knew I didn't want to be married, but I wasn't sure what I was supposed to do next. I had spent over two years with this person, we were in one another's lives and I didn't quite know how to just let that go, as it was the first real, long-term relationship that I had been in. Somewhere along the way, I had lost myself and I wasn't OK with that. I no longer trusted who I was as a person and often found myself conforming to a life that I wasn't 100% sure I wanted to lead.

After reading up on therapists that specialize on self-esteem and relationships, I made an appointment with Dr. G and on our first visit, I sat down, looked at her and started to cry. I hadn't even said hello. But I immediately felt comfortable in her space and I really needed to hear an opinion of someone who didn't know me or the situation that I was in. After about ten minutes of non-stop sobbing and nose-blowing, I looked up at her and said, "I'm actually a really funny person. I swear." She nodded, and it was then I first noticed her small frame and shoulder-length brown hair with bangs that swept to either side of her face, parted in the middle and I immediately realized that she reminded me of Joanna Gleason who played Miranda and Steve's therapist in the first *Sex and the City* movie. I had always wanted to have a Carrie moment during every woman's brief obsession with *Sex and the City*, too bad this wasn't it.

For the next year and a half, Dr. G helped me to get back on track with who I was and what I wanted out of relationships, not only with my ex-fiancé, who had been downgraded to my boyfriend (and eventually to nothing), but with all of my friends and family members. By the summer of 2010, I was back to my confident self when I got the news that I was sick. I called Dr. G for an emergency session. Having spent the majority of the week with my parents in

DC, around, all the time, I needed a break. I needed to see my trusty companion.

I walked into her office that August, sat down and said, "You are not going to believe this, I have cancer."

Her eyes opened wide, "WHAT! Are you kidding?"

"Nope. And you had just said how great I was doing." I laughed, since I had no tears left at this point.

At our previous session which had happened just before I left for Greece, we had talked about my progress over the past year and how great I was feeling. This would definitely be a set-back, to put it mildly.

"OK," she said slowly. "We can get through this."

"I cannot believe that I have cancer. Cancer! Who gets cancer at 32?" I asked her, shaking my head.

Dr. G shook hers in return, "I'm so sorry."

Dr. G and I spent the next hour talking about the diagnosis and how my parents had encroached in my space, and how I would be able to cope with the fact that they were going to be around a lot more in the upcoming year.

There are hundreds of online forums dedicated to any cancer you could ever imagine. There are groups for survivors, groups for terminal patients, groups for people who feel bad for people who are terminal. Support groups aside, we have become a world of groups and chatty Cathy's—just think of how much everyone shares on social media. And in most cases, I think it's great that everyone is so willing to share their story.

But I was not. I didn't want to sit in a group. I didn't want to create on online profile and commiserate with some woman in Kansas who was going through the same thing. I wanted Dr. G to help me navigate these new waters, even though she wasn't necessarily trained in how to cope with a cancer patient. She knew me, she knew what I had already been through, and she knew how I dealt with things and all that alone, for me, was a saving grace.

Together, we got through my diagnosis, my feelings of dread about treatment, my feelings of incompleteness after I learned that I would never look exactly like I used to, and most importantly, what to do with myself once I was better, which to many, can be the most difficult part of being handed a deck of cards like cancer and winning your hand.

Bottom line is this: you may not have a Dr. G in your life, and you may not even want one. But at some point, you will need to talk it out with someone that can either relate to your situation or someone who isn't as emotionally-invested as a close friend or family member. Express everything to them. Dump all of your BS into their office—it's what you're paying them for, anyway. I promise that you'll feel better afterwards.

Chapter 3: Saying Goodbye (September 2010)

September 21, 2010
Subject: Bye Bye

Boobies!
Tomorrow I shall undergo my transformation to become the ultimate bionic woman...I check into Sibley at 7:30am (who gets cut open that early???) and the surgery should take a few hours...Yes, I said hours. Then I'll be getting my groove back at Sibley.

I'd like to raise our glasses to say one last goodbye to the ladies. They've had a great run and have never let me down (well, except for the whole cancer thing). We spent a lot of fun nights around town, getting into hijinks and whatnot...so let's all have a moment for them :)

I bet you thought this was going to be one of those sad chapters about the later stages of cancer and having go say goodbye to loved ones and coping and all that other really depressing advice.

Nope.

I'm talking about saying goodbye to two very important body parts: my boobs. No matter how they've served you in the past, saying goodbye to one breast or two breasts is difficult. I mean, these are the girls that have been with you from the beginning. From the days when you wanted to pretend they weren't there, to the days when they got you out of parking tickets (or got you free drinks), to the time they got that cute boy in your freshman English lit class to finally look at you, your "assets" have played a pretty prominent role in your life.

Your breasts (or boobs, as I like to call them) are a part of you, so when your doctor tells you that they have to go, it's rough. When I first thought that I was only getting a chunk of my left breast removed, I wasn't happy but I was relieved that it was just a piece. No one would ever even notice, right? Well, that was before my second MRI which revealed another tumor just past the original culprit.

The news of my impending mastectomy was delivered to me over my lunch hour at the job I had just begun. (Of course, if you ask me now what I did for the three weeks I actually worked in that office, I couldn't tell you.) Starting a new job is hard enough without cancer: everything from finding your way around to trying to get rid of that new girl smell takes a pretty good amount of effort. Once you throw cancer into the mix, your mind will be in a million different places throughout the day. Not one of those places will be at your desk, on your computer, or in a meeting.

One day, as I was walking outside to take my lunch break, my phone rang. It was my mother. I had designated her as my health care liaison during the early days of my diagnosis, since I was still in the "cancer closet" with my new co-workers, trying to maintain some sense of normalcy at my new office. There was no way I could spend my days on the phone with a million different doctors in my makeshift cube with no real walls and a very sweet albeit inquisitive cube neighbor.

"Mer?" she asked as I was walking down L St. at noon, the streets crowded with businessmen and women.

"What? I'm going to grab lunch"

"They got the results back of your second MRI." She said in the tone that you know can lead to nothing positive.

"And…"

"They have to take the whole thing."

I stopped dead in my tracks right in front of the Potbelly sandwich shop on the corner of 19th and L and took a moment to process that sentence.

"No! Not happening." I yelled into the phone, tears welling up and making their way down my face. I could feel people on the street looking at me, wondering what I could have been so hysterical about. I wanted to be anywhere other than where I was at that moment.

"Mer, you don't have a choice. I got the name of a great plastic surgeon and we're going to make you an appointment."

By the time I had made it back to my apartment on 22nd and L, I was a complete mess. I had hung up on my mother because I could no longer deal with how rational she was being, and slid immediately into victim mode. It was as if I wanted her to validate my "Why me?" attitude, though now I realize that wouldn't have done me any good. I just felt desperate and helpless like a kid having a temper tantrum. I didn't want to lose my breast. It was part of who I was. Up until this point in my life, my 5'2 frame was supporting 34DD's (the size mainly due to being on birth control for almost five years). My boobs were nice. I had cleavage for days. Sure, my button downs usually required me to buy size larger, but my girls and I were a team. And now, we had to break up, and I was pissed.

I was so pissed that I was unwilling to take my mother's plastic surgeon recommendation. I stubbornly spent the rest of my day in my cubicle doing some research of my own, as I grumbled under my breath.

"What does she know about plastic surgeons in DC?" I thought, still begrudging my mom for being helpful. "She doesn't even LIVE here." While I was supposed to be studying my new employee handbook, I was on Google trying to figure out how to take advantage of this unfortunate and still unbelievable series of events—to see the "silver lining." And then, it happened. Somewhere in the middle of my meltdown, I had the following thought: This isn't a curse, it's an opportunity! Hear me out…

I'm *not* trying to convince you of some cheesy idea like, "When a door closes, a window opens." Because to be honest, everything about having to lose a part of your body is horrible and screws with your psyche. But let me keep it real for a second: when you get to 30 years old or so, your boobs start to get a little saggy. You can work out until the cows come home, but those girls will still get a little lower (and lower) each year. The best bras in the world can only hide it for so long. And so arrives the pseudo-silver lining: if you have to get your girls replaced because of breast cancer, your health insurance will be paying for most of it since it's not cosmetic. In other words, buck up, because you are getting new (relatively inexpensive) boobs!

Once I found my plastic surgeon, our first meeting was nerve-wracking. I had done my market research, being the marketing nerd that I am, but I was still scared about how much I didn't know. Though if you're wondering what market research looks like in the area of breasts, let me tell you this: marketing, my friends, is simply polling people to find out what they want. When it comes to asking individuals what they like and dislike when it comes to making purchases, people tend to voice strong opinions. And boobs, my friends, are no exception.

The first step is to define your target market. Since they're your boobs, you need to be honest and ask yourself this: who is really looking at them? Your girlfriends are good people to consult with, since true friends are the ones that will tell you when you look slutty or if you're teetering in the edge of slutty and party-classy.

Then, there are your gays and your guys (yes, even the ones you've never hooked up with). Let's be honest: if you have good guy friends, many of them are people you've either hooked up with or have hooked up with their friends at any given point in time. They see you on a regular basis and like it or not, the thought of seeing your boobs has probably crossed their minds if they're straight. If you're in a relationship, think of all this business as a gift to you and your partner: the gift of newer, perkier boobs, the boobs you had when you were 20. Ladies, this is possibly the only bonus of having breast cancer so it helps to embrace the positive.

Don't be shy! Ask detailed questions—the more specific the better! What size fits you best? Are you a B, but should be a C or a D? Are you a D but should be a B? Your plastic surgeon will tell you what they think, regardless of whether you ask. But at the end of the day, it's totally up to you: you hold the vision for the new girls.

Once you've decided what the new girls are going to look like, I recommend giving your original pair a proper sendoff. I've heard lots of stories about boob parties where women focus on celebrating their sense of liberation—they're glad to be rid of their boobs, and I say more power to them. Many women choose not to get reconstructive surgery, and I respect their choice 100%. But I knew that I was going to get new breasts, and that they were going to have to be pretty amazing. But before I could fully embrace this decision, I needed to say goodbye to the set that got me through the first 32 years of my life.

I know that lots of women will tell you to just do your thing and not worry about keeping other people in the loop. They may say, "It's not important what other people think of you," or "You don't need someone else to define you," particularly when it comes to the question of looks. Don't get me wrong: I'm all for being an independent woman and living one's own life, but I highly suggest giving your hard-working girls a proper party, preferably in one last really good night out. Get it all out at once—all the smoking, drinking, sleeping around, whatever it is you're into. I know that for most of our lives we're told that everything should be done in moderation, but in this case, I say, "Moderation, schmoderation." These are your breasts! Get out there and have some fun, because as much as I hate to break your stride, the next steps are nowhere nearly as fun.

In deciding who gets to be the last person to see, feel or fondle the girls, that is, of course up to you. Whether it's your boyfriend, husband, girlfriend, partner or just some random person that you happened to pick up around the way, the last person to touch them in a sexual capacity will be a memorable experience, because after this, that's it. Your next pair of breasts won't be the same as your original pair. They might be made of silicone or saline, or from fat taken from another part of your body. But whatever their new make-up, they aren't the ones you were born with. Despite my newfound level of excitement and acceptance, I found it extremely difficult to look in the mirror at the body that I had gotten to know so well over 32 years and think about the impending reality: that in just few weeks, I would look different. My anxiety had my head spinning with conjecture: I wondered what they would look like, if my next partner would be able to tell, how I would feel about them, what my friends would think. All of these thoughts are totally valid, even if they feel scary or uncomfortable. Accept your anxiety as it comes because it's natural, and fighting it won't help. No matter what your surgeons will tell you they will feel like or look like, you'll have no idea until that first time you take a good hard look at what you've been given.

I won't get into the details of my sendoff since I encourage you to go out and make your own memory. But I will say this: try to make it worthwhile. If you have already met your person, then make it as important as you would a birthday or anniversary. Choose your favorite restaurant, your favorite wine, whatever it is you like to do. And for single women, your great night could be one last great one night stand with a total stranger that you'll never see again, which also fun. (Just be careful because as I mentioned earlier, herpes is for life. Right now, you're dealing with a disease that's mostly curable.) And let me please note that you don't have to explain yourself, and anything you did or didn't do, to your oncologist. Their job is to make you better: they should not care what you do on the weekend, because that's what your therapist is for.

Out With the Old…In With the WHAT THE HELL JUST HAPPENED?!

Following my sendoff, I had more or less accepted the fact that I was about to undergo a pretty insane surgery that involved two surgeons and a whole mess of drugs. When my mother and I arrived at Sibley hospital on the morning of my surgery in September of 2010, I was in a total fog. Perhaps this was due to nerves, but I think it was largely due to the fact that it was the ridiculous hour of 7:00 AM. Plus, less than a month before, I was living a totally different life—one that definitely did not include surgery. Since I had never had an operation of any kind, I had absolutely no clue what I was in for. Sure, doctors will always try to walk you through the process of what they're going to be doing each step of the way. But their precision doesn't help to make things feel real. It's not until you are standing in the middle of a hospital room with nothing on but a gown and some hospital socks that the gravity of the situation sinks in.

As I waited for my surgery to get underway, I was repeatedly poked and prodded by various nurses who were taking blood samples, injecting an IV, and making sure I wasn't pregnant. I shuffled back and forth to my staging room nervously, wearing my starchy, itchy white and blue hospital gown. At one point, I found myself in the bowels of Sibley Hospital, close to the morgue I was sure, about to undergo yet another full body scan. I laid on the cold metal table, waiting for the scan to start and squeezed my eyes shut. "Maybe this is all a dream?" I thought. But when I opened my eyes, I was still on the table. Such was my luck.

As I waited for a nurse to escort me back to my staging room (because you cannot go ANYWHERE in a hospital unattended) I saw my chart casually sitting on a table, so of course, looked through it. It was my chart; I didn't see what the big deal was.

Here's a tip: hospitals take notes on you, much like some therapists do. As I quickly scoured the more than inch thick file with my name, I flipped through the notes I already knew. I had breast cancer. I was 32. I was single. Apparently, I was also, "educated and aware of my condition." I also learned that the Goldberg family as a whole was "open to learning and well-informed." I took this as a nice way of saying, "Here's a nice, educated Jewish family from New York, who has good health insurance." I remember feeling the desire to investigate my file further, but the nurse finally had returned and escorted me back to my staging room where the main event was rapidly approaching.

After about 15 minutes of pointless conversation with my mother, my plastic surgeon, Dr. B finally came in. I was ready to get the show on the road. I could tell that my mother was immediately smitten with Dr. B—his tall frame, good looks and gentle demeanor. I felt comfortable that they got along, but soon found myself more concerned with the fact that he was holding a Sharpie in his hand. He proceeded to use my torso as a own canvas, marking me up like a connect-the-dots activity book.

"What are you doing," I asked as he starting drawing on my skin?

"Just making marks so I know where I'm going," Dr. B reassured me. "Hey, you're belly button is a little off center," he added casually.

"What?"

"Don't worry, I'll fix it," he said circling the marker around my stomach.

While I was glad that Dr. B was so confident about the task at hand, my nerves kicked into full gear as the anesthesiologist walked in. "We have two types of anesthesia: strong and very strong. You're going to be getting the very strong."

Who was I to argue? I shook my head in understanding while trying to fight back the tears that were spontaneously springing to my eyes. This had been happening a lot since my diagnosis, I would just well-up at the drop of a hat. Part of me blamed it on the fact that I had stopped taking my birth control pills. In other words, my entire hormonal balance was different than it had been for years—and on top of that, I had cancer. For lack of a better word, I was a total mess.

The anesthesiologist smiled as he injected the cocktail into my arm and the last thing I remember was looking up at both Dr. P and Dr. B and saying, "Hey you guys? Don't fuck this up."

Seven hours later (or so I'm told), I slowly opened my eyes, wondering where the hell I was. What had just happened? What day was it? What time was it? Am I alive? I don't remember this room.

What room is this? I couldn't feel my hands and immediately wanted to rip the breathing tube out of my nose. My body felt numb, like my head wasn't attached. As I tried to lift my arm to remove the breathing tube, the nurses noticed that I had awoken and walked over to my bed.

"Hello. You're in recovery."

"Do I have a private room?" I asked. Note: the first question out of my mouth was *not* "Did it go well?" or "Is the cancer all gone?" or "How many lymph nodes did they take?" I can't explain why privacy was the first thing that occurred to me, but I can tell you that everything felt surreal.

The rest of the time I spent in recovery is pretty fuzzy to me now. Granted, I was on an insane amount of morphine, which, I'll add, is not so bad. But a short time later, things got clearer (and scarier), as they rolled me into my room, where I was finally able to take stock in what was going on under my hospital gown. I was hooked up to an IV for fluids and one for morphine, a catheter and a whole lot of bandages. My chest felt tight and there was a small black fanny-pack like sack around my neck. The fanny-pack held four drains that were connected to tubes running the length of my body, under my skin, that were meant to capture any fluid from both my new breast and my old one. I was a hot mess.

Since I had never spent any time in a hospital bed, I had no idea what to expect from my hospital stay. My mother, who refused to go back to my apartment (which I secretly really appreciated), moved into my room and slept on a pull out on the floor for the next three nights and four days as I laid in the bed next to her, wondering what was happening to my body.

On day two, I was awake for more than two hours and requested my Blackberry (I was still a Blackberry girl back then) only to realize that my hands were still numb from the copious amounts of anesthesia that I had received which freaked me out.

"Why can't I feel my hands?" I asked the nurse as she took my vitals.

"It's the anesthesia. It will go away eventually."

"Eventually? Awesome."

Nurses, as I learned, come in many shapes and sizes. Some are so nice that you never want them to leave, and some of them should not have graduated nursing school. On the third day after my surgery, I was informed that it was time for me to get out of bed. While I deeply wanted my life to return to a state of normalcy, I was exhausted, and the idea of trying to bounce back to reality was a notion that I was not ready to face. Put simply, I was still in a lot of physical pain and had no desire to use my energy to stand up from my hospital bed, which had since become my temporary command center. Even though I was somewhat homesick, I hadn't really even thought about getting up. I just kind of thought I'd be whisked away when it was time to go home. The idea of putting my two feet on the ground seemed like a foreign concept.

"No, thanks. I'll just stay here," I informed the nurse in an attempt to insert some humor into the conversation.

"You don't have a choice. You have to get up and start walking around." Note to self: not all nurses get, nor appreciate, sarcasm.

The idea of getting out of bed and moving scared me, which was a foreign feeling. What if I fell? What if my IV popped out? What if it really, *really* hurt?

But after an hour or so of prodding by the nurse, I finally got my legs to swing around the side of the bed (OK, the nurse helped too). And 20 minutes later, I was standing. This was definitely an out-of-body experience for me, since before this I had never had a surgery. In fact, I don't think I'd ever felt such intense limitations on what my body was able to do. I found this aspect incredibly frustrating, as many of you might. When you're in your 20s or 30s, there's very little the body *cannot* do; so the fact that it took me 20 minutes to get myself to stand up was disconcerting.

"OK, I'm standing. Can I sit now?"

"Try to walk around for a little," the nurse responded.

I clicked the morphine button and shuffled around the room, using my IV pole as a cane like a 90-year-old for a good two minutes before saying, "I think we've made some great progress here!" I was happy that I had not fallen, and was ready to get back into bed.

The following day, things felt the same—but this time, I had to go to the bathroom since my catheter had been removed. (I realized that taking away your catheter is their little trick to make you get up.) I didn't feel as triumphant as the previous day, and was having a harder time emotionally. My mother had finally agreed to go back to my apartment to shower; I was left with one of the weekend nurses, who was new to me, and not terribly friendly.

The new nurse eased me out of the bed to make sure I was standing on my own before watching me shuffle off to the bathroom. Due to the TRAM flap surgery, the middle of my body felt like Jell-O, weak and unstable. It was as if my entire body could unravel at any given moment. Though my body felt weak, my neck was still being weighed down by the fanny pack of drains, which hung around my neck and made me feel like a droopy Basset Hound. I used the IV pole as a crutch, lowering myself onto the toilet and then I realized that I could not get back up. The pain was so intense that I had no idea what to do.

"Hello?" I called out, expecting the nurse to come in and assist me. At this point, modesty had gone out the window. I figured these nurses had seen 90-year-olds completely naked, so my stitched up 32-year-old body would be a nice change for them.

Silence.

"Hello?" I called out again.

Nothing.

"Did she leave me in here? I think she left me in here!" I said to myself as I looked around like MacGuyver for any other props to help hoist me up so I could get out of the bathroom and start bashing some skulls.

"You can do this. Just get yourself up," I said to myself as I grasped the IV pole with both hands like a stripper, and pulled with all that I had in me to get myself out up and out.

Five minutes later, I had made it back to the bed and was able to lower myself to sit on the edge of the bed and repeatedly clicked the nurse button. When she finally came back into the room our conversation went something like this.

"Look at you! You got up all by yourself!" She exclaimed, proud of my accomplishment in a maternal kind of way. But she was not my mother, and I was not amused, nor did I feel particularly proud of myself.

"Was that a joke? You just leave people in there?" I asked. "Put me back into this bed, and close the door on your way out. And, never do that to me again," I told her sternly.

In this situation, I was definitely not being an exemplary patient. In fact, there were a few instances during my four-day stay at Sibley where I was less than gracious. Take it from me: you'll probably have times where you don't feel in the mood to be friendly either. If you want to be a bitch, do it. Let a parent, a boyfriend, a husband, a partner, a friend be the good cop. Let them bring the nurses coffee and apologize for your behavior. You have nothing to apologize for. You are classified as a "patient" in one form or another for the next year. You are no longer a visitor or just in for a quick procedure; you are under the care of numerous physicians and will be treated as such.

The next day, I was allowed to go home and I couldn't wait to have some privacy back in my own space again (even though "privacy" included living with my mother, who had temporarily moved into my studio apartment). We put an air mattress where a dining room table should've gone, and the couch nearby became my new command center.

On my first night home, I realized how badly I missed my adjustable hospital bed because laying down flat was simply not possible. Sure, I could stand at this point. I could even shuffle around to get from the couch to the kitchen. But sleeping? Forget about it. I spent two nights slumped down on my couch, using a chair as a footrest as Jeanee snored peacefully from my bed. I would throw things at her to make her stop and in the morning she would wake up surrounded by an array of books, DVD cases and tissues that I had intermittently thrown in her direction to get her to stop snoring. In between popping Oxycodone for the pain, my mother would chart and drain the small clear plastic bottles attached to my body to make sure that I was healing properly. She looked like a chemist, dumping out reddish-yellow liquid from these small containers that looked like mini-grenades. It was bizarre and surreal to realize that liquid was actually coming out of my body. Unable to deal with this horrific sight, I would keep my eyes closed, which was unusual for me, because I'm usually the one that can't look away.

Case and point. When Pleasance was pregnant with Saylor, she wanted to use a doula, which is a fancy word for a trained birthing coach. Without going for a full-fledge training, I volunteered to try on the doula role. I read a how-to book, packed a doula bag and off I went to the hospital with Pleasance and her husband Mel as soon as she went into labor. Mel and I joked around while Pleasance was resting in her bed, both nervous about the main event. When the time finally came, there we were, Mel on the left, me on the right, holding Pleasance's feet as she pushed Saylor out. Somewhere in between the pushing the doctor asked if I wanted to see the head and I was immediately unable to turn away from watching Saylor being expelled from Pleasance's womb. I couldn't avert my eyes so I found it strange that when it came to what was actually happening to my own body, I couldn't stand it, it made me cringe.

Clearly my unwillingness to accept what was happening to my own body was part of the whole denial stage of having cancer: you simply don't want to deal. But at this point, I was nowhere near the end of having to deal with the whole ordeal. Despite how much I felt like I'd already gone through, I was still just at the beginning, and was unprepared for such a long, involved process. No one ever warned me about how long-winded the treatment and recovery process can be—and even if they had, I'm not sure I would've understood. Intellectually, I knew that the body has an amazing capacity to recover if you just give it time. But really grasping the importance of patience was a notion that took me over a year to do. I just wanted everything to go back to the way it was as quickly as possible.

On my third day home post-surgery, it was time for my first field trip to Dr. B, my plastic surgeon so he could inspect his handwork. Since most of my body was still bandaged up, I had not actually seen myself in a week, which was strange since in the days leading up the surgery I was topless for most of the day while being inspected.

I stepped gingerly out of my apartment and down the step into Pleasance's car with my mother in the front seat, my fanny pack accessory still hanging from my neck. My body wanted so badly to sit upright and stretch, full of kinks from sleeping upright on the couch, but there was no way that I had the strength to make that happen just yet.

As we walked into Dr. B's office, I realized that I was now one of the women that I had been so intent on staring at during my first visit. I was officially a plastic surgery patient; I was someone who had *undergone* plastic surgery. This was still a concept that I was not able to wrap my head around. How was all of this possible? Take note: Oxycodone makes you think of some very strange things when you're seeing daylight and someone other than your mother for the first time in a week. I was convinced that the other women in the waiting room were now staring at me wondering what I had done as I stood in the waiting room, hair unwashed for days, in an oversized Goldberg the wrestler t-shirt and black sweatpants, unable to lower myself onto the plush leather couch in the waiting room.

"How are you doing?" he asked as he helped me to the reclining medical chair that was in the center of the exam room.

"You tell me," I said, striving for witty banter.

As he slowly pulled off the bandages I laid in the chair, my eyes squeezed shut, unable to look down at the mess of stitches, drains and bandages that temporarily covered my entire torso.

"Meredith, I need you to open your eyes so you can see what I'm showing you," he said.

I shook my head like a petulant child.

"Oh for Christ's sake, Meredith, just open your eyes," my mother called from the other side of the room.

I slowly opened my eyes and looked down. I looked like a robot with white tubes sticking out of four holes in my body. I immediately closed my eyes again. This was way harder to look at than Pleasance giving birth. This was happening to me and I hated it.

"Everything is healing nicely. The drain on the left side can come out today," he said as he reached for a pair of gloves.

"Wait, what?" I asked, still unprepared for any big changes, let alone for something to be removed from my body that I had just started getting used to. I assumed that the removal of the drains consisted of some sort of numbing medicine (or, at the very least, something topical). Nope. Nothing. He pulled that drain out and I felt it snake its way through my body. I'm not going to sugar coat how strange and uncomfortable this experience was because, put simply, it was horrible. If you are going to have to go through this, you're better off prepared, unlike I was. This drain in particular was affixed to my newly reconstructed left breast, and ran the length of my torso, ending just below my hipbone. The pain was intolerable. I winced and white knuckled the chair as he pulled it out and when he was done, I looked up at the good doctor and said, "Holy fuck that hurt like hell."

"Meredith. Language!" my mother scolded me. I shot her a look and she sat back down. Really? She was going to reprimand me for my language now?

I rolled my eyes at her and looked up at Dr. B as he began to further inspect. As he looked around, I did too, realizing that something wasn't quite right here. Something was missing....

"Umm, where's my nipple?" I asked, shocked.

"We discussed this. I took it off. You'll get a new one after you're done with all of your treatments."

"Oh." I replied, not wanting to admit that I had totally missed this part of the conversation. Of course, my facial expressions weren't hiding much: I was in shock. How could I have missed the part where he told me that I would be minus a nipple? I know exactly how I missed it now, looking back. I was so inundated with information that it clearly went in one ear and out the other, further proof that you need to have someone with you at these key appointments. Had I relented and let Chrys come with me for my initial meeting with Dr. B, I can guarantee you that I would not have been surprised to see my left breast sans nipple. The buddy system works people!

I looked down at the left side, which was now foreign to me. At 32, I was confronting the arrival of a new body part. Part of me almost wanted to say, "Nice to meet you" but I think that was most likely the pain medication talking. I took note of the stiches that ran across my breast, through the place where a nipple should be. My right side looked more familiar, smaller from the reduction that I had undergone to keep things as even as possible. Then, there was a ring of stitches around my remaining nipple.

Moving further down my body, I noticed another ring of stitches around my belly button and below that, a line of stitches that ran from left to right. My stomach was smooth and flat, a feat that I never could have accomplished without having all of the fat relocated to my left breast.

"Have you showered yet?" Dr. B asked as he was bandaging me back up.

"No," my mother interjected. I could not believe she had outed me. I was so scared to let water touch my reconstructed body that I was going through packages of baby wipes every day trying to get my body clean rather than just standing in the shower.

"Meredith, you have to shower."

I looked up at Dr. B hoping my sad, drug-induced blue eyes would diminish his stern words. No such luck.

"I know, I know," I lied. I had zero intention of getting into that shower until those drains were out of my body and I no longer looked like an alien. I didn't care how gross I was starting to look, never mind the dreadlocks that were starting to form in the back of my head. Even if I had wanted to shower, I couldn't lift my arms over my head to wash my hair.

It's a strange feeling not being able to trust your own body, but at this point, I really didn't. I thought that if I got into that shower, I would undoubtedly fall; after all, my body had betrayed me once, so why not again? I was scared that by some stupid accident, I'd cause even more harm to a body that has just gone through the ringer.

As I left Dr. B's office that day, I had one assignment to complete: take a shower and come back in a week so he could remove the rest of the drains. I shuffled out the door, past the women waiting for their chemical peels, and Jeanee and Pleasance took me for a well-deserved Starbucks before heading back home so I could resume my position on the couch, take another Oxy and a nap.

The next day, I reluctantly attempted my first shower, a welcome activity for the rest of my body. Unsure how to navigate this task, Jeanee asked if she could assist to which I replied, "Absolutely not." It was hard enough or me to grasp that my mother, the woman that I have not seriously depended upon physically since I was a teenager, was collecting body fluids like a chemist. There was no way I was letting her bathe me.

As I stood in the bathroom waiting to gather the courage to actually step into the shower, I stood there, naked, and cried. I hated that I couldn't trust myself enough to get into the shower, a task that I did every day up until that point. I hated that I looked like a rag doll, stitched and sewed in various places around my body. This was not the life that I was supposed to be living. I was supposed to be basking in my singledom, crushing it at my new job and enjoying my life. Never had I imagined that I'd be standing in my bathroom this weak and vulnerable. This is probably one of the times when your diagnosis will seem like the most unfair thing in the world, as if it were the karmic result of you pissing someone off in a former life. Even though this line of thinking may be irrational, allow yourself to have these moments. Allow yourself to stand naked in your bathroom, tears rolling down your face and onto your ridiculous fanny pack hanging around your neck. Allow yourself to feel sad and helpless. And when you think you're done freaking out, at least for the moment, just get in the shower. You will feel like a new person.

Chapter 4: The Dreaded Treatment (November 2010 – April 2011)

November 19, 2010
Subject: *Give me a C!*

Gimme a H!
Gimme an E!

OK...I've grown tired of this game...it spells chemo.

Just a quick little update from your old pal Mer to keep you in the loop on the next exciting chapter in what I like to call "Not Really Choosing Your Own Adventure"

I'm all set and ready to start my treatments.

I go in at 11am, leave at 3pm and then do it all again 3 weeks later. As for what happens in between, I have absolutely no idea...I've heard of people who were totally fine and go to work and run the world I've heard of people who had one round and was in bed until the next time...and I really, really hope that that isn't me. I'd settle for somewhere in the middle of all of that where I spend a day in bed feeling icky and then the rest of the time feeling like me, minus some hair, but hopefully most of it.

All joking aside...I know i make all this sound really fun and i know you're all really jealous but truth is...I'm fkng scared. This last part of getting better doesn't sound like fun, no matter how many Xanax or Percoset they give me. It just doesn't sound like something I want to do and if I could, I'd hide in some really fun country, just me and Port. But, if I'm not here to entertain you all, then who will????

Like most people that have never had cancer, I had no idea what chemotherapy was until I was sitting across from my oncologist talking about it. Sure, I had heard of it and knew that it was the course of treatment typically used to cure cancer, but where did it come from? Who invented it? I figured that since I had the time, I would find out all about these magical potions.

Turns out, the earliest forms of chemotherapy had been studied and tested in Europe by Louis Pasteur, Robert Koch, and Joseph Lister, in the early 19th century. Their work was followed by a student of Koch's, Paul Ehrlich who eventually went on to receive the Nobel Prize, for his studies of immunology and the chemical effect of paramidobenzol, phenylarsenoxyl, diamidoarsenobenzol, and pyocyanase on carcinomas and sarcomas. He summarized his observations in a book of 247 pages that is known to be the first book on chemotherapy before World War I.

After the First World War, studies of tumors and cancers moved overseas to the US, where national interest in curing cancer had been piqued. In 1937, the National Cancer Act was passed in Congress, followed by the creation of the American Cancer Society in 1946. From this point on, "modern chemotherapy" took over, leading us to today where there are several groups of chemotherapy and within each group are numerous variations.[7]

My main takeaway from the hours I spent Googling the history of chemotherapy goes something like this: tumors and carcinogens have always been treated with insanely technical and poisonous chemicals in order to kill the cancer cells. The chemicals are just mixed in such a way that they won't kill you, but just make everything in your body suffer.

I will never sugar coat my experience with chemotherapy to anyone who asks; it is not fun. It is tedious, frustrating, and, at times, will almost make you feel like you wish you were dead so you don't have to go through it anymore. It will also more than likely save your life.

After about six weeks after my surgery, I was up and mobile again meaning that I was ready to start treatment. Most of your doctors will want to make sure that you are fully healed from any surgery that you've had before they begin your chemotherapy adventure. Before I was given the okay to start my year of being poked, prodded and filled with chemicals, my oncologist wanted to make sure that my body could actually withstand chemotherapy and all that goes with it and scheduled me for a PET scan, CT scan and a ton of blood work. So many letters, what do they all mean! In medical terms, "a positron emission tomography (PET) scan is a unique type of imaging test that helps doctors see how the organs and tissues inside your body are actually functioning.

The test involves injecting a very small dose of a radioactive chemical, called a radiotracer, into the vein of your arm. Next, you will be asked to lie down on a flat examination table that is moved into the center of a PET scanner—a doughnut-like shaped machine. This machine detects and records the energy given off by the tracer substance and, with the aid of a computer, this energy is converted into three-dimensional pictures."[8]

In laymen's terms, the PET scan is done to make sure that there aren't any other parts of your body that are rotting from the inside. According to the MayoClinic's description, the CT scan "combines a series of X-ray views taken from many different angles to produce cross-sectional images of the bones and soft tissues inside your body." The individual images that are created help doctors get more information than they would with a plain X-ray. Or, in the words of the MayoClinic: "The resulting images can be compared to a loaf of sliced bread. Your doctor will be able to look at each of these slices individually or perform additional visualization to make 3-D images." [9]

    Essentially, these two tests are typically done before you start any course of chemotherapy to make sure that your body will in fact, be able to handle the hammer that is chemotherapy and that there isn't any other part of your system that has been affected by those pesky cancer cells. These tests all involve needles. Needles in your arm, needles in your hand, needles in your everything, and this is long before you've had a steady stream of chemotherapy coursing through your veins for any amount of time. Up until this point, most of us are used to getting blood drawn once every year or so. A quick FYI, in case it wasn't already clear: this will no longer be the case. You will have blood taken from you all the time from various nurses and doctors. Some of us, who are post-surgical and have had lymph nodes removed from any part of our bodies, are no longer allowed to have blood drawn from that side for fear of angering the remaining lymph nodes. Since I had gotten seven lymph nodes removed from my left side, my right side was now to bear the brunt of all needles. Some veins can handle this with the greatest of ease. Mine could not. By the third or fourth blood test post-surgery, all of the veins on my right side had revolted, leaving my arm bruised and sore.

On the day of my PET and CT scans, the nurses dug around on my right arm and hand until I was in tears. These tests both require different IV's. The PET scan IV requires a smaller needle while the CT scan one is a bit larger. My PET IV line went in just fine, but the CT line made me feel a pain like no other I'd ever experienced. When the nurses cannot find a vein, you'll know as soon as they try to push the saline into the vein. If it works, you immediately feel the cool saline rushing through your body and your mouth immediately takes on a metallic taste. If the nurse misses the vein, the saline runs wild in your body, burning your arm as a result. The first nurse eventually gave up and asked another nurse to come in for backup. After the second nurse had gone in twice at different points to no avail, I grabbed her hand and said, "Look. You have one more chance and then that's it. I will stay for the PET scan since I've already been prepped for it, but you can be the one to call my

Oncologist and tell him that no one here could find a vein." I was crying and made that poor nurse feel so bad I think she had tears in her eyes too.

After the PET/CT fiasco, I went to see Ari the Onco for the results of the PET, which had come back normal. Due to my age (and the fact that I was generally in good health, other than the cancer, of course), he agreed that I would not have to go back for another round of playing pincushion and I could forgo the CT scan, but he had one more delightful trick up his sleeve. He took one look at my right hand and arm and said, "There is no way that your veins are going to be able to handle a year of chemotherapy and testing. I'm recommending that you get a port before we start treatment."

"A what?" I asked, notebook out, pen in hand.

"A port. It's a small device that is placed under the skin and allows the nurses to access your veins without going through your arm every time. It will make your life much easier."

Easier. What a concept.

I told Ari the Onco, I'd set it up with my surgeon, and went home to do my due diligence on what the hell a port was. He insisted that a port can be done by anyone but I didn't trust "anyone," I wanted someone that already was familiar with the landscape that was my upper torso. I allowed myself to Google what a port was and tried my best not to actively search for Port-tastrophies. I settled on Wikipedia:

"A port consists of a reservoir compartment (the portal) that has a silicone bubble for needle insertion (the septum), with an attached plastic tube (the catheter). The device is surgically inserted under the skin in the upper chest or in the arm and appears as a bump under the skin. It requires no special maintenance and is completely internal so swimming and bathing are not a problem. The catheter runs from the portal and is surgically inserted into a vein (usually the jugular vein, subclavian vein, or superior vena cava). Ideally, the catheter terminates in the superior vena cava, just upstream of the right atrium. This position allows infused agents to be spread throughout the body quickly and efficiently." [10]

In other words, a port is a tiny piece of plastic that is under the skin that allows nurses to stick a needle right into your vein without having to search fastidiously, or make you use a stress ball.

While the thought of another surgery was daunting to me, this sounded like a really good idea, especially in the state I was in after all the bruising. Back in the day, ports were large and cumbersome and stuck out of your body so you looked like an alien. You also had to make sure they were continually flushed and cleaned. Today, ports are tiny and leave only a small scar on your chest and on the side of your neck. They're hardly visible.

The procedure for getting a port is an in-and-out surgery that takes only about an hour. Of course, there is the rigmarole that comes with any hospital surgery, a process that I was unfortunately familiar with. There was the starchy, itchy robe and ridiculous looking socks with tread on the bottom, there was the thousand questions and the inserting of the IV, which the nurse at the hospital was able to do with ease.

"Hey, she found a vein, looks like I don't need to be here," I said, as I jokingly went to walk out the door.

My mother and father were un-amused. They had both made the journey from NY to DC for this procedure and once again did not seem to appreciate my attempts at levity.

"Meredith, does everything have to be a joke with you?" my mother asked.

"I learned it by watching you," I responded, feeling my Xanax kick in. I felt as calm and collected as someone who was about to be put under for the second time in three months could be.

I said goodbye to my parents, waving like a contestant on Miss America as they wheeled me into the operating room where I was met with the familiar face of Dr. P.

"Don't screw this up either," I said. About five seconds later, I was out cold and Port was in.

I like to refer to Port in the third person because it's just funnier that way. After all, there really is nothing funny about having a piece of plastic inserted into your body. When I woke up after the surgery, I looked at the bandaged area and thought to myself, "Great, how long will it be until I shower again." So far, having cancer was making me into one dirty bird.

The good news: port surgery is nowhere near as invasive as any kind of surgery that you've already been subjected to so your bounce back time is a lot faster. Before you know it, you and your Port will be getting to know one another, going for trips and showing him/her around town. The bad news: before you know it, you'll be cleared by your doctors for your first round of chemotherapy.

The Truth About Chemotherapy

Everyone's chemotherapy treatment is different; it's one of the great snowflakes of cancer, if you will. The treatment is dependent on what is driving your cancer. For breast cancer there are essentially three driving forces, or what are called "receptors": estrogen, progesterone and HER2/neu, which is a human epidermal receptor. Each one is used to pinpoint the type of breast cancer you have and how it is going to be treated.

The type of breast cancer that I was diagnosed with is DCIS, AKA the most common type of non-invasive breast cancer. What this means is that the cancer cells are inside the ducts, but have not spread through the walls of the ducts into the surrounding breast tissue. Basically, this meant that the cancer had not spread and was contained to my left breast, which was "great news" according to all of my doctors. Every time I heard this, I'd silently reply, "Great news for you maybe." No matter how much your doctors will sympathize with you, they'll never *really* get what you're going through. Once I accepted this fact (early on, fortunately), I was able to let go a little bit.

When they biopsy your special little tumor, they will not only be able to tell you what type of cancer you have, but will also check to see which of the three receptors are positive (or not if breast cancer is what you're packin'). Your chemotherapy will be crafted according to your results. You could go blind reading about the numerous types of cancer drugs that are available and many doctors will offer you a chance to go on a medical trial. I cannot speak to this since I didn't want to try one and Ari the Onco seemed pretty sure that he had the magic combination to get me back to my former glory.

The Talk

I had numerous meltdowns during my diagnosis, surgery, treatment, post-treatment phases and you probably will, too. Honestly, it's better if you just accept the fact that from time to time you will, at any given point of any doctor's appointment, cry, heave, sob, have your nose run down your face, drool a little, and just generally lose your shit. You think you're being a child about it, but in reality, no one expects you to be stoic all of the time even though that path may seem virtuous. I was along that path as well for about a day until I realized that I couldn't hold back the feelings of anger and helplessness. It helps if you accept these uncomfortable feelings, remembering that the discomfort will pass. Eventually, you will be able to separate yourself from the tough feelings, and one day you *may* even be able to laugh at them. But no rush, that's down the road.

You will be faced with an obscene amount of information during visits to all of your doctors. Some of it will make sense, most of it won't. Sometimes you'll pay attention, most of the time, you'll have some song playing over and over in your head or making a mental list of things to do, but there are times when you are listening so intently that you could snap a pencil with your mind. For me, there were those crucial few moments when I was listening to my doctors or nurses and I just knew I was about to have a meltdown. The most memorable instance of this happened when I met with Ari the Onco two weeks after my surgery in early October to talk about my impending treatment, and the all of the wonderful side effects that were going to accompany it.

See, I don't know about everyone else out there, but cancer didn't make me feel sick. I felt and looked fine and other than the dark circles under my eyes and the acute phase of pain I felt during my recovery time from surgery. The problem with traditional treatments for cancer, like chemotherapy, is that they make most people feel horrible for the entire length of their treatment. This is the reason why many people make the effort to avoid chemotherapy at all costs, which I completely understand. But I just wanted to get better. ASAP.

During the initial stages of my diagnosis, the biopsy and subsequent testing revealed that my tumor was estrogen and HER2/neu positive meaning that the way to cure my cancer was going to be pretty targeted. I receive another "good news" line from my doctors. But none of this is good news, it's just news. Good news would have come in August after my first biopsy had come back negative. Nothing since then had been good news.

The treatment that I was going to be handed was a cocktail of three different drugs: Taxotere, Carboplatin and Herceptin (TCH). Each comes in its own special IV bag and is clear like water (or vodka, as I had often dreamed). Taxotere, or Docetaxel, is used alone or in combination with other medications to treat certain types of breast, lung, prostate, stomach, and head and neck cancers. Docetaxel injection is in a class of medications called taxanes. It works by stopping the growth and spread of cancer cells.[11]

The side effects of Taxotere are listed as, but not limited to: nausea, vomiting, diarrhea, constipation, changes in taste, extreme tiredness, muscle, joint, or bone pain, hair loss, nail changes, increased eye tearing, sores in the mouth and throat, redness, dryness, or swelling at the site where the medication was injected.

Carboplatin is an anticancer ("antineoplastic" or "cytotoxic") chemotherapy drug. Carboplatin is classified as an "alkylating agent" that is used to treat ovarian cancer as well as lung, head and neck, endometrial, esophageal, bladder, breast, and cervical cancers; central nervous system or germ cell tumors; osteogenic sarcoma. It's also used during the preparation treatment for a stem cell or bone marrow transplant. Side effects of this wonder drug are listed as: low blood counts (including red blood cells, white blood cells and platelets), Nadir (meaning low point, nadir is the point in time between chemotherapy cycles in which you experience low blood counts), nausea and vomiting usually occurring within 24 hours of treatment, taste changes, hair loss, weakness and an abnormal magnesium level.[12]

Taking notes on the side effects? You should because both of these drugs that are designed to kill anything in their paths pack quite a wallop to your entire body.

Herceptin is a newer drug on the market that was created to specifically attack the HER2/neu receptor, which they didn't have up until a few years ago. To quote the eponymous website Herceptin.com, "Herceptin is approved for the treatment of early-stage breast cancer that is Human Epidermal growth factor Receptor 2-positive (HER2+) and has spread into the lymph nodes, or is HER2-positive and has not spread into the lymph nodes." Herceptin can be used in different ways, combined with different drugs. According to Herceptin.com, there are multiple ways to use the drug:

1. "As part of a treatment course including the chemotherapy drugs doxorubicin, cyclophosphamide, and either paclitaxel or docetaxel. This treatment course is known as "AC→TH."
2. With the chemotherapy drugs docetaxel and carboplatin. This treatment course is known as "TCH."
3. Alone after treatment with multiple other therapies, including an anthracycline (doxorubicin)-based therapy (a type of chemotherapy)."[13]

Herceptin has no side effects, which was nice to hear since the laundry list of things side effects of the Taxotere and Carboplatin are enough to send someone hiding under the bed (or a fit of hysterics. Either or).

While I had been scheduled to undergo six rounds of this magical combination, which came out to about six months, I was also told that once the course of TCH had been completed, I still had another six months of Herceptin-only treatments, so I was basically looking at a year of being hooked up to an IV every 21 days, if you're keeping track.

So there I sat, in Ari the Onco's office, finally ready to ask the question that all women who are about to undergo chemo are wont to ask: "Will I lose my hair?"

"We'll go over all of the possible side effects with T, the head oncology nurse once we're done here. She'll show you around the treatment area and answer any questions about the drugs," he said, dismissing my question.

I thought to myself, "Did he just glaze over my question and kind of ignore me? Fuck me, I'm going to lose my hair."

Up until the hair question, cancer is something that you can pretty much hide from the outside world. But hair is external. People see our hair. I know that my friends have been making fun of my giant Jew-fro since college, when I first obtained the nickname "the Dark Helmet". My light-brown hair is wavy and often appears GIANT. In other words, there's A LOT of it, so if it were to, oh, I don't know, FALL OUT, people would certainly notice. People would stare. And I knew that implied in the stare would be the accompanying question, "What's wrong with her? Don't you think she's too young for cancer?" And I'll be honest: you'll probably get those looks. Try as hard as you might to avoid it, but you will probably even get this look from family and friends. You will get this look from nurses at your doctors' offices and from the people in the waiting room, since most of them will be considerably older than you are and on occasion, you will even get this look from your doctors and if you're like me, then you will not like it.

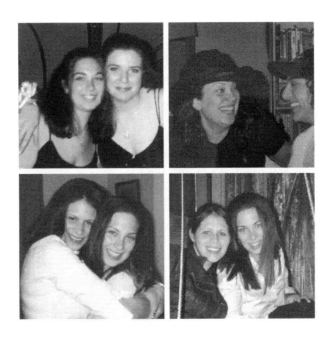

The dark helmet in its many iterations.

Ari the Onco pressed on about the mechanics behind TCH after clearly dismissing my very important question but he had already lost me at that point. All I could think about was my hair and you will too, it's really hard not to. There's nothing okay with the idea of losing your hair. I don't care how many women say it's empowering, it's not; it's a bullshit side effect from a bullshit disease.

When he was finally finished with his TCH talk, he lead me back to the treatment room for a tour of the facilities so I would have some idea of what the treatment area looked like. There are different types of places where you can receive treatment, whether that be in your doctor's office, a hospital or separate, private facility. I was going to be receiving treatment in his office, which was a smaller facility in a private office, which I preferred for two reasons. The first: it was three blocks from my apartment, meaning that my back-and-forth journey wouldn't require me to use public transportation or cabs. The second was that I felt that I would receive a more personalized treatment in a smaller facility. Some patients are OK remaining a name and an insurance card; I am not one of the people. If I am going to be spending an inordinate amount of time in one place, then I want the people around me to know who I am. I didn't just want to be "patient X."

The nurses in the office decorate the treatment room like it's a pediatrician's office. There is a bowl of candy and decorations for every holiday from Christmas to St. Patrick's Day. The treatment room is arranged in sort of a semi-circle of treatment chairs, each with their own IV machine that is used to dispense each magical potion. The chairs are designed to look like barcaloungers but I assure you are nowhere near as comfortable as your dad's favorite chair. They're made out of a pleather-y material and are in various shades of medical greys, mauves and blues that are reminiscent of the 1970's, the dreariness exacerbated by the antiseptic fluorescent lighting. I definitely give the nurses credit for trying to make it look like a place you'd want to spend time. But there's no denying the reality that it's depressing and sad, and the minute you step in that office, you want to go home.

 As I looked around I secretly clicked my heels together to see if it would work and wisk me away to anywhere but there. But I had no such luck. I eased myself into one of the treatment chairs that wasn't in use by a patient and was introduced to T, my oncology nurse and ruler of all things treatment-related. Tough-talking and no-nonsense, T was in her mid-50's with a short bob of strawberry blonde hair and a southern accent. Her pink scrubs adorned with cartoon characters did nothing to hide her harsh demeanor. She was a personality and we didn't exactly hit it off. T sat me down and began to explain the side effects that would soon consume my life. She brought out a pink notebook that the drug company clearly created in a veiled attempt to soften the blow of the medicines they've created to "cure" us. I took one look at the book and looked up at T, "You're kidding me with this, right?" T is definitely not a pink diary kind of woman. She has a "don't mess with me" aura, even though she was a very present force in the room. Right off the bat, I knew that working with her would involve feeling well taken care of, yet mildly frightened by her gruffness. She continued on trying to sell me on this pink atrocity that I'm sure you will be assaulted with as well. I was slowly yet surely getting really sick of the color pink.

"Here, these are stickers to help you chart how you're feeling."

I looked down at the smiley and frowny faced stickers and looked back up at her. Remember that meltdown I was telling you about? This pushed it from possibly avoidable to most likely going to happen.

"If I feel like shit, I'm going to tell you I feel like shit. I'm not going to put a sticker in that book."

I could see T's face take a step back to register what had just spewed out of my mouth. I was going to be one of "those" patients. In her mind, I was going to be difficult. In mine, I was just responding the way any normal girl would respond to smiley face stickers.

Enough of this sticker stuff; I was ready to get down to business. "Will I lose my hair?" I asked again after I had safely stuffed my new pink sticker book in my bag along with all of my other breast cancer reading materials that I had no desire to read.

"Yes."

I looked at T and nodded to indicate understanding. And then it happened—the immediate welling of the eyes, shortness of breath, hands sweating, nose running and the final collapse of any social functionality. I was crying hard in the treatment room with a woman who already hates me, which of course made my cry harder. My body shook in the chair as T rubbed my arm and said, "You're going to be okay." But in that moment, I didn't think that was true and in all honesty, neither will you. Nothing about hearing all of the terrible things that are about to happen to you and your body will make you feel comforted.

I don't remember the rest of that conversation or the appointment for that matter, but I can tell you it ended shortly thereafter since once Ari the Onco re-emerged he could tell that I was at my max capacity and backed off. Ask your doctors to do the same. It will save you a lot of wasted time repeating the same information over and over again that you missed when you were in overload mode.

I bawled as I walked the three blocks back to my apartment and once I was home I took a long look at myself in the mirror, trying to imagine what I would look like without any hair. "Who even knows what the shape of my head looked like?" I wondered, freaked out. You'll ask something similar, I'm sure. I mean, how many of us EVER really thought about what the shapes of our head are other than in the 90's when Sinead O'Connor's big old bald head was in our face.

Dealing with the notion of losing one's hair is a big deal. We've all met women who have faced cancer head on, rocking out pink wigs, G.I. Jane hair and we've all applauded them for that. But then it happens to you, and you realize that your own head is going to be bald. Something changes, something clicks. Maybe this is the point where certain women say, "I'm going to rock this" and some say, "I really don't want to do this." Or a variation thereof.

For me, this was inarguably the second reaction: a "I REALLY, REALLY don't want to do this" kind of moment. I started going down the "why me" "this sucks" "fuck everyone" emotional spiral as we all have once or twice. After about a week of feel victimized, frustrated, and insanely pissed off, I finally started to climb out of the funk. I asked Pleasance to take me to the wig store to try on some styles so we could see what I was about to be dealing with.

Armed with a Xanax and the prescription that had been written for me for a prosthetic wig, I went to the wig store. I thought I was going to be OK, as if trying on wigs is the same thing as trying on dresses. But no: it's a surreal experience. You may get the feeling that you're in a place that you're not supposed to be, almost as if you forget where you are and why. I will say that most of the people you will come in contact with at wig stores are typically trained to engage with women and men in times of an illness, and are generally helpful and super nice. No, this doesn't soften the blow, but it does help…a little.

I can see why some women can embrace the whole wig thing; it's a chance to try out something new—a new color or new style without having to really commit to the look for very long. I had a brief moment where I thought, "This could be fun" and then I tried a wig on. I chose a look that was not so far off from my style at the time (save for the fact that it was pin straight, a feat that I could never reach without the help of Japanese chemicals and a flat iron), and the saleswoman helped me place the wig on my head correctly.

"How will this stay on my head with all this hair underneath?" I thought to myself. Then it hit me: there wouldn't be any hair underneath. There would be nothing. I was going to be bald.

By the time she was done placing the wig, my heart was racing and I was one step away from full-on panic attack. Turning to look in the mirror was, for lack of a better word, weird. I looked like the Hasidic Jewish version of me; all I needed was a skirt covering my knees and a long-sleeved shirt to cover my elbows and there I was, super Jew Mer. I turned to Pleasance and Saylor, "Do you like it?"

Both shook their heads.

"Yep, me neither." I ripped the wig off and realized that I didn't even want to try another style or color. I wanted to keep my hair and look like me. Some of you will feel this way and some of you will love the whole process. It's not a matter of being braver than others; it's just a matter of personal preference and how to deal with a really shitty situation.

We drove home after the wig debacle of 2010. I tried to be upbeat and jovial about the excursion, but I felt helpless and angry. There had to be another way. And if not, then there had to be a better wig store. And *then* a funny thing happened.

Frozen Vanity

My first cousin Barrie had been diagnosed with breast cancer around the same time I was. After she and I had heard the news about one other, we started emailing to exchange stories. Our family dynamic is the stuff that soap operas are made of—cheating, fighting, backstabbing and lying. Given that I'm the youngest grandchild out of six, I was a relative child when most of the bad stuff was going down, though it all came to a head at my bat mitzvah in 1991. In summary, there was an all-out brawl on the dance floor, which lives only on VHS tape and our minds. To this day, I cannot hear the Caribbean-resort hit, "Hand's Up" without going into some sort of PTSD state in which my eyes widen, and the song must be turned off immediately.

Due to our age difference (about 16 years), Barrie and I we were never that close, so reaching out to her was strange to me. Add to the mix that we had went from being part of a pretty dysfunctional family that still spent time together often to being part of a *totally* dysfunctional family that never hung out unless someone died. So for she and I to share our experiences about something as personal an illness (which we both quickly found out ran through our genetics) was at first a bit awkward. As it turned out, most of my female cousins and my aunt on my maternal side carried the BRAC gene, my mother and I the only two who were spared.

Barrie and I lived in two different worlds for most of my life. Her father (AKA my uncle, my mother's brother), benefitted from our family's business, which my grandfather started when he immigrated to the United States from Russia with two of his 18 brothers and sisters. When my uncle took over for my grandfather, he subsequently pushed my mother out of the family business, leaving us as the "have-nots. Over time, however, Barrie had blazed her own trail and now lived out of the fray with her family out on Long Island.

At this point, I was post-surgery, pre-chemotherapy but still in the cancer-closet to most people outside of my inner circle. Barrie was in the same position. My reasoning was pretty simple: I was not 100% ready for the pity look that I was eventually going to get from everyone, and I wasn't ready to field the steady stream of questions from people that weren't close to me. In particular, I did not want my ex-fiancé finding out. Our ending had not been particularly kind or mature. It consisted of him hurling Polish curses at me while drunk, telling me that no one would ever love me again, in the same breath as he asked me why I didn't love him anymore. He was eventually escorted out of my apartment, and out of my life, and I liked it that way. I was not ready to reveal my story to anyone that could have gotten the information back to him. I never questioned why Barrie hadn't been telling people; I just understood and accepted it for what it was. As it turned out, we were both similar in that we had both grown to be quiet women, not having our business out in the streets, a trait that was pretty familiar to my extended family for years.

    She had been doing some research of her own and had come across a rather new-to-the-U.S. hair conservation therapy called Penguin Cold Cap Therapy. The science of it is based on a pretty simple idea; if you keep your head at a certain temperature (-31 degrees Celsius, or 23.8 degrees Fahrenheit) all of the blood supply is cut off to your hair follicles, preventing the drugs from reaching your head, keeping your hair intact. At the time that I learned about the caps, not many people were using this as part of their chemotherapy, mainly because it hadn't been fully approved by the FDA. But once I heard about what it could do, I was sold. The more I read, the more I knew that I was willing to do anything to make this happen for me. I envisioned myself being able to live the life I was living before I found out that I was sick and felt an immediate sense of empowerment. All of a sudden, cancer, chemotherapy and everything that was going to come with it, seemed far more manageable. As both Barrie and I navigated our treatment plans, she found out that she would not have to undergo chemotherapy yet had already began a dialogue with The Rapunzel Project, a non-profit organization created in order to help cancer treatment facilities get the freezers needed in order to keep the caps at a constant temperature when they are being used.

The cost at the time to have a freezer delivered to any doctor's facility was $1,500, plus the cost of shipping a 6' freezer from the middle of the country. My cousin had become pretty entrenched in learning about this fascinating technology, and what it meant for women going through this process. The Rapunzel Project and extended an offer to help me, by arranging to have a freezer delivered to my oncologist's office and renting me the caps needed for the length of my treatment. Since my chemotherapy was going to be four hours long, every 21 days for six rounds and the caps needed to be switched out every 30 minutes, it was recommended that I rent 12 caps. This meant a $600.00 deposit in addition to the cost of renting the caps—$500.00 a month.

When my cousin first told me that she was going to cover the cost for me to utilize this treatment, I was shocked. While Barrie and I are blood related, I had little to no interaction with her for about 20 years. The cynical part of me wondered if her act of insane kindness would come back to bite me in the ass one day. (After all, this was the case with most of my family's events in life: everything came at a price, and good deeds never went unpunished. I wasn't sure if I was in a place to deal with that.) Since Barrie's father, my uncle, had passed away from cancer about a year prior, I had come to terms with the fact that I would never really have the family dynamic that I always wanted, and was beginning to be OK with that. I had felt that I had formed my own family in DC and they were amazing enough that I didn't necessarily miss the big family Passover meals that I grew up with as a child. I finally felt safe with the deep connections and sense of community I'd made for myself, so opening up to accept such an amazing gift from Barrie felt risky. It was as if being able to receive her generosity meant that I'd be making myself vulnerable to receive more pain and disappointment from people that I had been hurt and disappointed by for most of my life.

After talking it over with my therapist, Dr. G, I came to the realization that I needed to not let my fears and insecurities run my decision-making, and that I could be OK with accepting this gift. That said, there was still one more major hurdle emotional to overcome in addition to accepting Barrie's generosity: nurse T.

When I approached Ari the Onco with the idea he said, "As long as it's legal I don't care what you try on the side." T was another story.

"That won't work," nurse T said to me in a matter-of-fact, somewhat cold tone. I got the sense that she felt threatened by me in some way, as if I was trying to change things in her universe. She ruled the chemotherapy roost and I was trying to change it up.

"Well, I want to try," I explained. She didn't want to hear more of it.

As my relationship with T grew more and more tense each day that inched closer to the beginning of my treatment, I found myself in an unfamiliar emotional landscape: one in which I was not necessarily conflict averse. Let me explain: throughout my life, I've never been one to engage in confrontation. In fact, I usually avoid it at all costs. Historically, when I am upset about a situation, I avoid confronting it, and instead let it fester. The typical result is that the resentment, anger or whatever it is manifests itself for me physically—whether that be knots in my stomach for days or back pain or jitters. Note: I'm not proud of this approach, but it's how I've always been. Yet in this situation, things felt different. Perhaps it was a survival mechanism at work, but I didn't have energy to let stomach knots build up. I knew I had to deal with my nurse T-related issues head on.

The more I went back and forth with T about trying this conservation therapy, the more I started to question myself. I noticed my vanity, and also took notice of how much I wanted to control the situation, one, which was so far outside of my control.

With regard to the question of vanity, I've never really thought of myself as a particularly vain person. Sure, I like to look good when I go out, but I've never spent more than 30 minutes to get ready for anything and you'll never find me getting a blow out every week; hell, before this I could go for days without washing my hair.

With regard to the question of control, I've never realized how much the act of *trying* to control a situation can really mess with your psyche, especially when that situation involves an illness like cancer. We've all led lives that we probably think of, on some level, as a series of actions and experiences that result from choices that we've made. That is, up until our diagnosis. We are able to "control" where we live, who we love, what we eat and so on. So when that fundamental sense of control is taken away by the news of a disease, it can be quite jarring to say the least. I noticed that I was searching desperately for any way to perceive the situation in a way that gave me a sense of control. Sure, I had chosen the doctors who were going to be treating me, but that wasn't enough. Hair conservation therapy would allow me to control a larger aspect of cancer and as much work and stress as it added to my life, I was willing to do whatever it took to maintain some sense of normalcy over the next year and if this technology worked like it's said to, then I would have control over some part of the experience. No, I wouldn't be able to control the nausea or the exhaustion or what the disease would do or not do next. But if I could take the steps to ensure that I looked the same way I always have, then that was a fight I was willing to engage in, for better or for worse.

After about two weeks of back and forth between me and T, the Rapunzel Project team, my cousin and my mother, nurse T was finally able to relent and accept the 6' freezer to be used first, by me and then, ideally by anyone who wanted to use the cold caps going forward. The goal of the freezer was to be one of the first in Washington, DC, a story that was guaranteed to bring notice to the small K Street practice, a notion that no one at the office seemed comfortable with and that was fine with me. I was perfectly content keeping the news about the freezer contained to the practice as long as I was permitted to use them and they worked.

I didn't even read the possible side effects of the caps, of which there are many, as there are with any product that is new to the market. There was a chance it wouldn't work. There was a chance that should have the cancer spread to my brain the chemotherapy would not reach my brain, allowing any mets to grow. There was a chance the freezing wouldn't work at all and I would have sat with a frozen head for a combined total of 48 hours (six treatments, eight hours of freezing). But with all of the negatives, there was one positive: this was a way for me to possibly retain some shred of dignity during this horrible ordeal. That was all I needed to know.

Using Penguin Cold Cap Therapy for hair conservation is not only a commitment for the patient. It's a team effort, one that my team, which consisted of all of my friends and family were ready to take part in. The caps look like individual Smurf-blue ice turbans and weigh about five pounds each. The come in their own little plastic container houses and are strapped onto the head with a series of Velcro flaps and bands.

When it finally came time to start my first treatment, the 220v freezer that had been sent to my oncologist's office had been so strong that when it was installed, it blew all of the circuits in the office causing the backup generator to turn on, on a Friday afternoon, while there were other patients receiving their treatment. Nurse T was not amused; my mother sent a fruit basked as an apology. While we were waiting for our new, less extreme 115v freezer to arrive, we were using two 50 pound Coleman coolers, that most people use for tailgating, packed with dry ice that was being transported to and from my oncologist's office, by me and my parents. Remember when I said I chose my oncologist in part because of his proximity to my apartment? This logic came in handy as the three of us trekked down K St. in the middle, DC, during rush hour with coolers full of the caps and dry ice weighing in at probably about 100 lbs. each.

The first time you go in for treatment is really scary. You're likely going to be the youngest person in the doctor's office, and you are usually going to be in a room with other patients who are receiving a variety of infusions and transfusions. Whatever it is, none of it is fun. I know that some of you have visions of best friends laughing and sucking down rainbow colored popsicles, having their own private party. These are lies. Yes, your friends can come and sit with you, but it's not a party and you are not going to want to be in any semblance of a sun dress and/or stiletto. My advice to you: get yourself some really comfortable clothes and a giant blanket.

    The whole first treatment experience is akin to your first day of classes in college or the first day at a new job. You don't know where anything is, you don't know anyone and it feels like there's a secret club that you aren't a part of. But of course, you aren't there to make friends. As I said before, cancer is a full time job—so think of chemotherapy as your on-the-job training. You will see these people for as long as you are in treatment and then, ideally you will never have to see them again. Long story short? If you don't feel like making friends and bonding over the fact that you are all strapped to an IV machine, and you just want to bury your head in your phone, it's OK, you have every right to be cagey and in your own world.

One would think that a four-hour infusion every 21 days would be quite enough, but no, there's more. In addition to the chemotherapy, many doctors will have you take a steroid the day before, day of and day after your treatment to prevent any type of allergic reaction to the chemotherapy. This was fun, because in addition to being anxious before each treatment, especially your first, you will not be able to sleep! Hooray! You will lie in your bed, some of you alone, some of you with a loved one, some of you with your parents on the floor on an air mattress, snoring away while you lay awake, flipping channels and wondering what the hell was going to happen the next day.

I remember on the first day of my treatment, I rolled out of bed, having been awake for hours already, not fully being able to grasp where I was going. It was a week before Thanksgiving and the plan went something like this: get the treatment so that the next day I could go home with my parents for Thanksgiving in Long Island. Of course, we had no idea how I was going to feel. Exhausted? Unable to hold anything down? Depressed? I felt totally ignorant about how my body would react to the beating it was about to take, and that scared me to no end.

After an arduous 10-minute hike up K Street with our two coolers full of dry ice and the caps, we arrived at my oncologist's office looking like a travelling circus. My father and I were both in sweats, my mother in jeans and sneakers schlepping my bag of tricks which included my phone, two books, a magazine and a giant yellow blanket to keep my body warm as my head was reduced to -31 degrees. As we waited for the show to begin, my mother paced back and forth while my father meticulously read over the directions again and again as they are pretty specific. Twenty minutes before treatment begins (the "pre-med" stage, during which you get your IV going and take some Tylenol and a hit of Benadryl), one cap was to be placed on your head for 20 minutes and the cap had to be at exactly -31 degrees Celsius. After 20 minutes, the treatment has begun, although the caps then need to be switched out every 30 minutes, ideally within a specific two-minute window. While we had our infrared thermometer to track the temperature of the caps and special gloves to handle the dry ice, we had no idea what we were doing.

Before you are taken back to the treatment room, you have to have a vial of blood drawn so the doctors can chart your counts of red blood cells, white blood cells and a whole bunch of other three letter acronyms that I never understood. They will also take your blood pressure. On this first day, mine was unusually high.

"I can't imagine why my blood pressure is like this?" I questioned facetiously, my words dripping with sarcasm.

"You'll be OK, dear," the nurse reassured me in her Jamaican accent that I grew to find quite comforting over the next several months. From there, I was shuffled back to the treatment room where my parents were waiting with my coolers of caps. There was also nurse T, looking less than thrilled at the set-up we had going on in the corner of the room. Once I had gotten myself settled, I began affixing moleskin to my forehead to avoid freezer burn on my head and ears. Not only was I about to strap a five-pound blue cap on my head but I was also covered in moleskin, a product typically used to protect my feet from my 4" stilettos.

With the moleskin plastering my head and ears and the pre-meds flowing into Port, the first cap was ready to be placed on my head. We fumbled with the first cap and took almost five minutes to get it directly onto my head. My father and I had done two or three dry runs before the actual treatment, but now add in the fact that the caps were now below freezing and not as pliable as they were when we did our test runs. Needless to say, it took a while to get it right. The tighter my father pulled the cap, the closer it got to my scalp and the cold set in. A chill immediately ran down from the top of my head to the bottom of my feet and my hands turned to ice. I love cold, don't get me wrong. My friends always call my apartment the igloo due to the fact that I keep it at a constant 60 degrees. But this? This was a cold I had never experienced before. The -31 degree cap laughed at my sweatpants, sweater, Uggs and blanket as the cold penetrated every layer of clothing I had on. I knew then that this was not going to be easy.

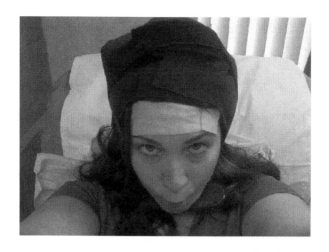

Round 1. Also, ready to tell your fortune.

In addition to the fact that I was absolutely frozen to the bone, I looked ridiculous. I felt other patients staring at me, wondering what the hell I was doing and I wondered as the pre-med stage ended and nurse T attached the first bag of toxic medicine that began coursing through my body. "What if this doesn't work? What if I do all of this and I still end up bald?" The panic began to set in as I felt my freezing cold hands turn warm and clammy. Was this a huge waste of time and money? Was I being ridiculous to try a therapy that wasn't 100% proven? These last few thoughts swirled around my mind as the Benadryl finally overpowered me and I was out cold, only to be awoken 30 minutes later by my father

"Time to change the cap."

I groggily opened my eyes as my father began pulling the Velcro straps off the cap to remove it and replace it with another as my mother directed. I sat back in the lounge chair wincing as the Velcro straps that are used to tighten the caps became a snarled mess in my hair, ripping out chunks of my hair before the treatment had even ended.

"Be careful!" I yelled like a hair dictator, unable to control my anger due to the steroids.

During the first treatment (and after we had changed the cap two or three times), my father and I found a good rhythm, which also included my mother who had been put in charge of getting me soup or anything that could keep me warm as I tried to get in as many quick 20 minute naps as possible in-between cap changes. Times when I had to get up to use the bathroom in-between bags of medicine, I would catch a glimpse of the other patients, sitting in their chairs, sleeping or reading quietly, yet there I was walking around with a giant blue ice turban on my head. "What was I thinking?" I would ask myself as I'd look in the mirror in the bathroom before returning to my chair to continue the arduous process of chemotherapy. There was something absurd about it all. I just had to laugh.

This process continued for the four hours of chemo, and then for an additional four hours once we returned to my apartment. You can only imagine the stares I received from people walking past me on the street, my bright blue cap covered by a hoodie and a scarf, making my head look about 10x bigger than it really is. Once we arrived home, the fun *really* began. With no strangers looking or nurses to contend with, my frustration, anger and sheer exhaustion became overwhelming. I would shout profanities at an alarming rate that immediately made me guilty as soon as they left my mouth.

My parents did not sign up for this, they never asked for a child who was going to need them more at 32 than they had at 18 and although I was angry at my father for pulling my hair, I was extremely grateful at the same time. Those two thoughts combined made tears spring to my eyes on a daily basis. I never wanted to think about the alternative, but the questions often flooded my mind;

What if my parent's didn't have the means to help me? What if my cousin had never found out about the caps and I was just sitting around waiting for all of my hair to fall out? What if she hadn't offered to pay for it? What if I didn't have any family at all? What if I had gotten married and I was stuck with someone who my parents didn't love; would they still have come and helped?

If you are fortunate enough to have these people in your life, and especially if they step up in any of the ways that I had experienced, then you, like me will learn to be eternally grateful for them. Note: your family members will still probably remain the people that drive you craziest in life.

We finally finished switching the caps out at about 8:30 p.m. that night and by the end I was beyond exhausted yet dutifully took another steroid before lying awake in bed wondering what the next day was going to feel like. "Would I start throwing up soon? Would all of my hair fall out? Would I be too tired to leave the apartment?" These were all questions that filled my mind for the duration of the day.

I woke up the next morning feeling fine. I was fine. I wasn't tired or nauseous. My head wasn't throbbing and I wasn't running to the bathroom every five minutes or needing to take the anti-nausea medication, Compazine that had been prescribed. I thought to myself, "This is it? This isn't so bad. I can do this." It was with this mentality that I was ready to make the trip home with my parents on Amtrak back to New York. As the day wore on and we barreled our way to Long Island, I began to feel tired, but nothing out of the ordinary—just as tired as anyone would be who had just been on steroids for three days and on a complete emotional rollercoaster.

I remember getting home to my house on Long Island and resting on the couch. I was tired but fatigue was still my only symptom. And then Thanksgiving came.

Thanksgiving has never been my favorite food holiday. I mean, sure I get into eating turkey and stuffing as part of the tradition, but I've never really salivated in anticipation of the meal itself. Taking my typical indifference with all the emotional trauma into account, I wasn't particularly surprised when the meal rolled around and I wasn't super excited to eat. I looked at my plate and decided on a bite of turkey dipped in gravy. As I chewed my first bite, it tasted like a mix of pepper and metal, as if someone had dropped a canister of pepper into the gravy by accident. Thinking that it was just that bite, I moved onto the scoop of stuffing that sat just to the left of the turkey. Pepper/metal once again.

"Does this taste weird to you guys?" I asked my parents and cousins that sat around me at the table. It was just five of us total, a quiet holiday for a change, no one really wanting to make the effort to cook since we had been in DC for the earlier part of the week.

"No, does it taste weird to you?" my mother responded. Normally she would have been offended that I was questioning her cooking since my mother is a beast in the kitchen, but everyone at the table just kind of looked at me sympathetically, almost like they were waiting for my head to spin around.

"It tastes peppery," I remarked as I gradually realized that I was beginning to feel the effects of my treatment. The peppery taste in my mouth intensified even without food in my mouth, and I was beginning to feel queasy. I was definitely not hungry and all of a sudden a wave of exhaustion overcame me that I had not felt since I had mononucleosis in 9th grade.

"I'm sorry. I need to go lie down," I explained further as I put down my fork and with my eyes half closed. I walked from the dining room to the den, where I fell onto the couch and remained there for the next two days. I could feel my parents watching me make my way into the den, wondering if this was the tip of some kind of chemotherapy iceberg and that it would all be downhill from here. I wondered, as I fell asleep if I was going to feel this way forever.

Exhaustion from chemotherapy is a kind of fatigue that consumes you in a way you've never felt consumed. It's like having the flu on top of a hangover on top of mono, some of which may be unfamiliar to you. Put simply: you will be insanely tired and no amount of rest will give you the energy you want back. My most prominent symptom was this paralyzing fatigue, but other odd symptoms cropped up. Water started tasting weird, for instance, almost like my mouth had a film on it.

Everyone's reaction to chemo is different and mine seemed to result in three main symptoms: exhaustion, weird food tastes and an aversion to spice, something that I had always prided myself on. I soon found comfort in three foods in particular that I continued to eat during the course of my treatment; frozen yogurt (the real tangy kind), cantaloupe and smoked salmon. To drink, I would typically have green tea or whole fruit smoothies. To answer the question you're probably asking: yes, going through chemotherapy is akin to being pregnant, at least from what I've heard about pregnancy. Certain foods taste totally amazing and others make you want to gag. Through all the changes that my body was experiencing with tiredness and taste changes, I was also waiting to see what was going to happen with my hair.

Many cancer patients will often begin to lose their hair 14 days after their first treatment. I counted down the days. I slept on a satin pillowcase, as instructed by the Rapunzel Project and the handful of women that had gone through this process before me. I didn't wash my hair for four days after treatment, and then out of fear, I waited few more days, waiting, wondering if the theory of simply freezing my head would keep the toxic chemicals from having it all fall out.

Waiting for your hair to fall out is a daunting task that begins first thing in the morning when you jump out of bed and examine your pillow for any hairs that may have escaped overnight. This process continues all day—staring at the back of your shirt when you take it off, inspecting your coat or scarf or any article of clothing you may have been wearing that day. Trips to visit friends ended up being a scavenger hunt on their couch to see if I had left any strands behind.

About a week and half after my first treatment, I finally worked up the courage to wash it. I gingerly applied the suggested shampoo and just kind of stood there in the shower wondering how to wash it out without running my fingers through my head. After careful deliberation, I just stood under the stream of lukewarm water, hoping for the best and praying that if this treatment worked I would have to end up getting my head shaved anyway due to the mats were accumulating in the back of my head like my dog used to get. As soon as the water touched my head, I turned around to inspect the drain and the hair catcher that I had been made to get my building's super years ago due to the fact that I have always been a massive shedder and would more often than not clog the drain.

There were a few more strands than usual, but nothing out of the ordinary. I blinked to make sure my eyes weren't just playing tricks on me. They weren't. The caps had worked for the first round. I breathed a large sigh, one that I seemed to have been holding in since the treatment and continued to rinse the shampoo out of my hair.

When I stepped out of the shower and began to spray the leave-in conditioner in my hair again, as suggested by the Rapunzel Project, I stared into my bathroom mirror and made a deal with my hair.

"OK, you stay in and I will never dry, color or chemically straighten you again. Promise."

I carefully ran my fingers through sections of my hair, forgoing a comb, and ended this routine by gently wrapping my hair around a metal-less hair tie. Clips, headbands or anything that would pull or damage my hair were off-limits for the next few months as was using any product. Thankfully this wasn't happening in the summer, as humidity is disastrous for my giant head of hair. I've been using some kind of "hair tamer" since I was a teenager to prevent the Dark Helmet from emerging (especially in the warmer months). But now, my hair would have to go au-naturel, not like it mattered what I looked like anyway since I didn't leave the house much, which leads me to another wonderful side effect of chemotherapy.

Your Body Will Reject You

During the first few weeks in-between my first and second treatments, I learned a valuable lesson about chemotherapy and your immune system. Your immune system will reject you repeatedly. That is, every time you step foot around another person, you will get sick.

On my way back from New York after Thanksgiving I had enough energy to make it from Long Island to Penn Station and then from Penn Station to Union Station back in DC. But somewhere between Trenton and Dover, I started to feel sick, and not like nauseous chemo sick, like sneezing, aching, fever sick. As I crawled into bed that night, my entire head felt like it was a balloon. Luckily, I had to check in with Ari the Onco the next day for follow up blood work where we discovered that my little jaunt to New York resulted in a white count that was almost at zero.

Nurse T sat me down and said, "You're nutropenic. I'm going to need you to stay home for the next few days. No metro, no crowds, no children, no super markets. If you need to go anywhere, you have to wear a mask and we're going to need to give you two Nuopgen shots, one today, one tomorrow."

"What's nutropenic?" I asked, blowing my nose for the thousandth time that day as I envisioned myself as a prisoner in my own home for the next few days. I laughed as I put the surgical mask in my bag. There was no way I was going to step foot outside with that thing on as my friends and I had always made fun of people who walked down the street wearing masks. Karma.

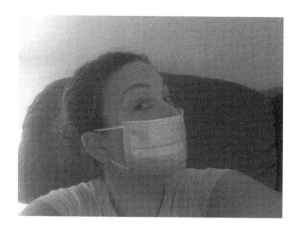

Confined to my apartment, post round 1.

For those of you who have not yet experienced receiving Nupogen or being nutropenic here's a quick rundown from the handy-dandy MayoClinic: "Neutropenia is an abnormally low count of neutrophils, white blood cells that help your immune system fight off infections. The lower your neutrophil count, the more vulnerable you are to infectious diseases."[14]

Basically: while your body is fighting with every inch of its being to kill whatever cancer may or may not be still floating around in your body, the drugs you are getting to help you fight the cancer is also killing all of your white blood cells in the process.

To combat the wallop that the drugs do to your system and your white counts, science created Nupogen, (filgrastim) which is a man-made form of a protein that stimulates the growth of white blood cells in your body to help fight against infection. Basically, it's a shot, but not like any old shot, it's a super shot that is designed to go right into your bone marrow to help produce new white blood cells.

I was in no way prepared for the pain that this shot would cause, and once again, found myself hurling profanities in the middle of yet another doctor's office. As I practiced the yoga breathing techniques that Pleasance had taught me, I also found myself yelling "Holy Fuck" along with some of my exhales. So much for being zen.

As I walked around the block home from Ari the Onco's office, my body felt like it was slowly being drowned in cement. I had wanted to stop and get some soup on the way but decided that my Ugg'd feet would not be able to make it the extra block. I came home, closed the door and fell onto the couch where I once again remained for the next week.

I have no idea what is in Nupogen or how it makes others feel but here's an explanation of its effect on my system. The following morning I woke up feeling like my eyes had become dirty windows overnight. Everything looked foggy and furry and my entire body felt heavy and Jello-y. I had no desire to return to Ari the Onco's office for the second shot of Nupogen; I was almost sure that they were trying to kill me, but I dutifully made it to my appointment. When I showed up in leggings, Uggs, a giant hoodie and a scarf, my blue eyes surrounded by dark circles, nurse T looked at me quizzically, and someone concerned.

"You don't look so good," she remarked.

"I feel like shit. What did you do to me?" I replied, now completely devoid of the impulse to be polite.

"It's the Nupogen," she said, as I unzipped my sweater, ready to endure another shot.

"Ready?" nurse T asked as I squeezed my eyes shut and took a deep breath in.

The long thin needle penetrated my skin and I could feel my body falling deeper into a level of tired that I didn't know existed. Once again, I dragged my weak body back home and got into bed.

Unfortunately, Nupogen became part of my chemotherapy routine. A day after treatment, I would come back to the office for one shot, and then another one 24 hours later. This was followed up with a week of "dirty window eyes" on my couch with the remote. I binged on all of the series I had been meaning to catch up like *The Wire, Friday Night Lights* and *Freaks and Geeks*. I would try to read, but my eyes always had trouble focusing and my brain could not retain information from one page to the next. It was like reading Groundhog Day over and over, in other words, fruitless. This is another wonderful little side effect of chemotherapy called Chemo Brain. There have been lots of studies as to whether this condition really exists or not, and I will tell you it does. It is not a made up thing like unicorns or big foot.

According to the American Cancer Society, "Research has shown that some chemotherapy agents can cause certain kinds of changes in the brain. Though the brain usually recovers over time, the sometimes vague yet distressing mental changes cancer patients notice are real, not imagined. These changes can make people unable to go back to their school, work, or social activities, or make it so that it takes a lot of mental effort to do so." [15]

For some people, Chemo Brain comes in the form of short-term memory loss, trouble concentrating, trouble multi-tasking or slower recall. I had read about Chemo Brain shortly after I had started treatment and had asked my oncologist about it. He didn't discount it, but didn't seem completely convinced that it really existed. "No way is that going to happen to me," I thought to myself. Fast forward to New Year's Eve, when I was about three treatments in and was feeling well enough to surround myself with a small group of good friends to ring in 2011.

As we watched the pre-ball drop shows on TV someone asked who a certain performer was on the screen.

"Oh, that's…" I started to say, but couldn't remember. "That's….what's her name? Shit. What is her name? I know who that is, why can I not remember her name?"

I could see this performer's face and I could see the name of the performer in my mind, but could not for the life of me put the two together to complete the sentence.

"Are you drunk?" Chrys asked me, unable to believe that I, the queen of pop cultural trivia, could not name the singer on the television.

"Chemo Brain," I said, bowing and shaking my head in shame.

"It'll come back to you," she replied.

I wondered if she was right about that. As I progressed through my treatment, I started noticing that I was most definitely experiencing some brain-related side-effects of the treatment. For me, Chemo Brain had a consistent manifestation: I would start a sentence and then totally lose my train of thought half way. I would start a task and then forget about it moments later, and finally, and most depressing to me, I just didn't get the jokes as quickly as I normally would. It feels like your brain has been suspended in time and your reactions move at a glacial pace. My once quick wit was relegated to a slow wit; my usual snappy retorts had been replaced with regular glazed-over looks of confusion.

The good news is that chemo brain gets better…eventually. In the meantime, here are a few quick tips that helped me keep my brain from totally becoming mush during and after treatment.

- **Put down the Candy Crush.** There's no doubt that you'll have a lot of time in waiting rooms. Any chance you get to ask your brain if it's on, do it. Instead of playing mindless iPhone games, try a crossword puzzle or Soduku, or really any type of activity that requires you to use your brain to think logically.
- **Keep your schedule**. You may be tired all the time, but try, if you can to wake up and go to sleep at the same time every day. Your body will like the schedule and can help you from getting all out of sorts. If you aren't working, this is also a good way to keep your body from going into shock when you do eventually return to work

- **Write it down!** Again, you'll have the time to keep yourself organized. Try using online reminders or planners. I found that making a "to-do" list every morning helped, because at times by noon, I had forgotten what I needed to do that day and would find myself standing in the middle of the street wondering, "where am I going again?"

- **Walk it out.** Take a walk, do some light yoga, do whatever it is that your body can handle. Moderate exercise can help with stress, fatigue and depression, all factors that can exacerbate Chemo Brain.

- **Let yourself take naps.** Lovely, wonderful naps. Rest your body, rest your mind and the two will appreciate the gesture.[16]

About three to four months post-chemotherapy, I noticed that I was remembering things better, but from time to time I would still forget what I was saying mid-sentence and as much as I would love to tell you that years later I was completely back to normal, I'm not, and while it might not be noticeable to people around me, I can feel it. I often forget the word that I want to use and will stare at my computer for minutes before the word I was searching for appears in front of me. The same thing will happen in conversations with friends, family and even worst, during more pressured interactions like meetings at work. I find myself stumbling on my words from time to time, sounding like a complete moron, especially when I am speaking quickly or having a discussion with a co-worker and I'm trying to explain a strategy or a thought that I'm having. I've found that the best way to backtrack is to stop talking, give my brain my minute to catch up to my mouth and then begin again.

The Waiting Game

Whether it's sitting at in the waiting room, biding your time until your next treatment, waiting for your hair to fall out, or simply waiting to feel better or worse from chemotherapy, you will find that you spend a whole lot of time waiting. Just waiting.

For many of us going through chemotherapy, there are actually days when you feel OK. You will wake up on these days saying to yourself, "Hey, I feel not-terrible right now." You may then wonder how long that will last. But while you're waiting for feel worse again you might want to take that time to get out of the house. On days when I was feeling not bad, not great, but well enough, I liked to try to act like a functioning member of society. This typically happened about a week after each series of Nupogen shots. I was ready to get out of the house for a little and re-join the world as my white counts came back up to a respectable level. During my "well" days, I dipped my toe into the real world with a walk around the block or spending time with friends and on occasion, receiving work from the company I had started with before my diagnosis. Since legally they couldn't fire me, they gave me enough work to keep me busy and allowed me to work from home. I'd go into the office for meetings if I felt up to it, and I'd wonder how long I would be able to sit in a meeting before I wanted to take a nap. The waiting game never ended, with one exception as I made it through my second and then third round of chemotherapy. My hair.

By the time my third round of chemo, the halfway point had arrived. Sometime in January 2011, my oncologist finally took notice of the fact that I was not bald. The TCH should have left me bald two after my first treatment, yet there I sat, eyebrows thinning, eyelashes falling out, no hair on my arms or legs, but a full head of crazy, wavy, albeit a tad dirty, brown hair.

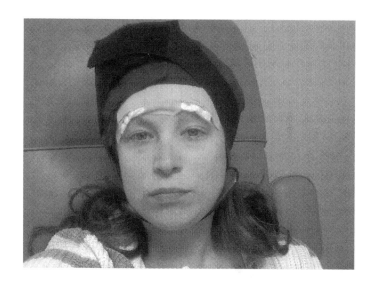

Round 3. Brow-less, but a full head of har.

"You seem to still have all of your hair," he said during my routine pre-chemotherapy exam. This was the first time that he had acknowledged the fact that I was even using the caps since he had distanced himself from the initial back and forth that my family and I had with nurse T when we were trying to get approval to use the therapy.

"Yes," I replied with a smile, although what I really wanted to say was, "SEE, I TOLD YOU IT WOULD WORK!"

"Very interesting," he responded nonchalantly.

Of course, he wouldn't have noticed that I had lost a significant amount of hair, but by no means enough for anyone to actually notice. The only reason I knew how much hair I was losing was because I was the one who saw it collecting in my shower. But other than the few thousand strands that I didn't really need anyway, my hair was perfectly in place and I was no longer waiting for the hair-shoe to drop.

Sure, I had developed permanent dark rings around my eyes and my entire being was puffy from the steroids and chemotherapy, but my hair remained intact all through treatment.

I'm sure that there are many of you that see hair conservation as a ridiculous addition of stress to an already stressful situation and I agree with that sentiment. It's a lot of work, it's a lot of added pain and it's a lot of added help. I would do it again in a nanosecond. For me, the ability to maintain my sense of self, even if it was somewhat based in vanity, was critical in maintaining a sense of normalcy during my chemo.

There's something about being able to maintain any kind of control in a situation that most people have zero control over that's really empowering. It allowed me to avoid the looks, the stares, the points and the pity look from total strangers. It allowed me to enjoy my "well" days with friends. It allowed me to go to dinners without feeling too self-conscious; while I might not have been able to taste or digest a lot of what I was eating, the fact that I could do it without anyone looking over me was all I needed to power through the rest of my treatments.

If your first day of chemotherapy is like your first day of school, then your last day of chemotherapy is like the last day of senior year of high school. Just like wandering the halls saying goodbye to all of your teachers and friends with an air of survival and pride, you will walk through the doctor's office with an unprecedented sense of relief. And you'll see the newbies, getting ready for their first treatment, looking lost and confused and scared and all you want to do is hug them and say, "It will be OK." But you stop yourself, because you remember that you weren't ready to hear that when it was your first day.

My last TCH treatment was in April of 2011, and while I still had another six months of Herceptin treatments that would be bringing me back to the oncologist every 21 days, there was levity to my last treatment that I felt as my parents and I walked into the office. My mother and father would no longer need to make the trip to DC every month and set up camp on my living room floor. While I still had a few more hills to climb with regards to treatment, I had made it through what had been, up until that point, the hardest part. I survived the toxic onslaught of chemicals swirling through me.

As I prepped myself for my final four hours of chemotherapy, I noticed how mechanical my routine had become: sit in the waiting room, get blood pressure checked, get blood work, meet with Ari the Onco, walk down the hall to where the private treatment room was, cover my head and ears in moleskin, wrap myself in a blanket as my father put the first cap on my head, pre-meds flowing in my body followed by an hour of Taxotere, hour of

Carboplatin and an hour of Herceptin, my body succumbing to the Benadryl in 20 minute cat naps.

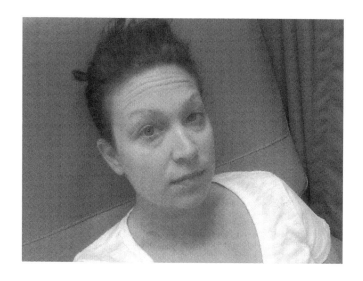

Taken the day of my last TCH treatment. Six rounds, no eyebrows, no eyelashes, but a full head of hair.

At the end of the final treatment, as my parents and I began to collect our things, nurse T and the other nurses came into the room and began blowing bubbles in celebration. In addition to my relief, it felt amazing to know that over time, nurse T had become an advocate for me, always making sure that the private treatment room was reserved for me, making sure I had a fun Band-Aid to lift my spirits after each treatment or Nupogen shot and protecting the freezer from being damaged and ensuring it remained running while it wasn't in use. Nurse T was now my buddy, and after seeing the amazing results of the Penguin Cold Cap Therapy, she actually wanted to keep the freezer even though I no longer needed it. Since Herceptin has no side effects and does not cause hair loss, my need for the caps had come to an end. My 12 Smurf blue turbans could be packed up and sent back so another woman could begin her process.

The freezer, we had hoped would stay at my oncologist's office for other people to use, but the other oncologist in the practice would not allow his patients to use Penguin Cold Cap Therapy due to its "unproven effectiveness" (all he had to do was take one look at me as proof) but he had his reasons and neither I nor Nurse T could change his mind.

Today, the freezer lives at another practice in Washington, DC where they were more than thrilled to be able to offer this to their patients. As more and more women and men have begun to use Penguin Cold Cap Therapy, I can only wonder if the other oncologist thinks twice about this "unproven" treatment.

After going through six, four-hour treatments, the hour-long Herceptin-only treatments were like a cake walk. The routine remained the same, minus the added stress of the cold caps and since it was only an hour and I had already been receiving this medicine for six months, I no longer had to get Benadryl, allowing me to cheerfully sit and relax for an hour, read a book, g-chat with my friends and get the scoop from the nurses on what's been going on in their lives. It was almost like going to the salon. OK, not really, but I didn't mind it. It, like chemo, just became part of my routine.

My final Herceptin treatment was right before Thanksgiving 2011, almost a year to the date of my first chemotherapy treatment in November 2010. The feeling was similar to the last round of chemotherapy, but with a lot less jubilation in the office. I had already survived the hard part, so Herceptin was the easy stuff, the in-and-out stuff. I finished my last hour of Herceptin, said my "see you laters" to the nurses and stepped out into the warm fall day and walked home wondering if I had done it all.

Had I been cured?

Chapter 5: You're Positively Radiating! (April 2011 – June 2011)

March 29, 2011

Subject: Radiating with Mer

I most certainly am not done with my journey down Cancer Road...Oh no, my friends, the chemo and the continued Herceptin treatments are just a warm up for the next journey I like call: "Radiating With Mer"

Yes. It will be a show I'm hosting for six weeks at GW, EVERY DAY for about a half hour. I'll be in the studio taking your calls about how to radiate in a number of capacities. How to radiate heat, b/c I'll apparently get a really weird and horrible sunburn right on my shoulder area (which if you have ever seen me in the summer, you all know that I am the queen of the random tan/burn). How to radiate lying still for 30 mins every day so they don't zap the wrong part of the body. I mean, I donno about you, but any time a doc says there's a small chance we can radiate your heart since it's on the left side, well that just makes you feel all warm and fuzzy (mind you, this is a 1 in 5,000 chance)

On "Radiate With Mer" we can also talk about how to radiate exhaustion since that's what a lot of people say they feel afterwards...I just can't tell you how excited I am to find out what's in my bag of radiation tricks!

I've been dealing (or perhaps not dealing) with this last bit of radiation news over the past two weeks. And to say that it's dampened my spirit is kind of an understatement. Just what I wanted right before my birthday: a GIANT RANDOM SUNBURN on my neck. So hot! It really sucks to walk into a doctor's office with the glimmer of hope that you have avoided radiation, only to find out from your team of doctors that it had already been decided a long time ago that this was always in the cards for you. I mean really just fk it up. But you learn to rationalize with yourself...if I do this now, I'll never have to do it again.

Radiation, or as I like to call it "radiating" (I find that every word is more fun if you make it into a verb) is often going to accompany to your cancer journey or the one stop shop. It's true that it's less invasive than chemotherapy, but it is just as annoying; most people who are subjected to radiation have to go every weekday for a certain period of time.

I didn't find a radiation oncologist until I was just about finished with chemotherapy in April of 2011. Ari the Onco had always tried to reassure me by putting off conversations about radiation. "We'll talk about radiation down the road," he would say often. So unsurprisingly, when the road appeared, I was a little shell-shocked since I hadn't been expecting it at a particular time. As I walked into the radiation oncologist's office, I thought I was there as a formality, just to talk to her about options. I quickly learned that this was not the case. Ari the Onco had recommended a woman named Dr. H, who was a small, impeccably-dressed and beautiful

Indian woman no older than 45. Dr. H was based out of Sibley Hospital, where I had had my surgery eight months prior.

As I said, I wasn't prepared for the fact that I was going to need radiation. When I walked back into Sibley Hospital to meet with Dr. H, it was vaguely traumatic. Just being there reminded me of my surgery, and gave me slight chills of fear even though nothing was happening.

But despite my chills, I still found myself in somewhat of a state of denial. As I made my way to the cancer center, I foolishly had some of the same mindset that I had going into my first sonogram before I had been diagnosed: "I'm just here for a routine visit, I'll be in and out in a little while, I have things to do," I said to myself, rationalizing my discomfort away with avoidance. So when Dr. H started talking to me about scheduling matters during our discussion, I was, to say the least, pretty confused.

"What do you mean I *have* to have radiation? I thought that this was a possibility," I asked as I studied her face for answers. I was trying really, really hard not to cry in yet another doctor's office.

"Meredith, this was always in the cards for you. With three positive lymph nodes and the degree of the cancer that you had, you don't really have a choice."

I took a deep breath in and exhaled slowly. This was the first time that anyone had told me that my cancer had been severe. For more than six months, I had been living with a relatively casual mindset about my situation, even in the moments where I was most scared. "Oh I have cancer, no big deal," I'd think to myself on some level. This moment was the first time I felt fully in touch with the fact that this wasn't the case at all. Staring at Dr. H amidst this realization, my eyes began to fill up and my palms grew clammy and cold.

"I don't understand," I said, tears streaming down my face. "I thought that after the chemo it was only six more Herceptin treatments. No one told me that radiation was a definite."

Dr. H took my hand. "I'm so sorry," she said, trying her best to comfort me in a decidedly uncomfortable situation. "I wish this was over for you too so you can get back to your life, but you have to have six weeks of radiation."

She went onto explain further what the reasoning was behind my needing radiation. While the mastectomy removed the cancer and the chemotherapy killed whatever was still lurking, there was still a chance that something else was out there festering in my body. She also explained that the radiation would cut the chance of anything recurring by 85%, which was admittedly comforting. While the thought of putting my body through any additional torture was heartbreaking, I knew that it was either deal with it then or deal with it years down the road, but at the time six weeks seemed like a lifetime when I had just spent six months exhausted on my couch.

"SIX WEEKS?!" I yelled, my eyes practically bugging out of my head.

"Yes, every Monday through Friday for six weeks. The whole process takes about 20 minutes. You'll be in and out each time very quickly."

"Six weeks!" I repeated, unable to grasp what was happening.

As Dr. H rubbed my arm as I sobbed in her office, she tried to go over how radiation works.

"You go in, you lie down, you get the radiation, you go home and go about your day."

Easy for her to say. She wasn't the one that had to do it.

"Side effects?" I asked. I had, at this point, become a seasoned patient, asking as many questions as possible and no longer caring about how much time I took talking to each doctor.

"It can feel and look like a bad sunburn around the area of radiation. Some people feel tired. Some people don't feel anything."

"Awesome," I replied sarcastically.

"I'm sorry that you have to go through this and I know that you thought you were finished, but I promise that it won't be as bad as chemotherapy."

When our conversation turned from, "let's talk about radiation" to "let's schedule radiation," I found myself dreading the commute as much as the radiation itself. My mind filled with thoughts of schlepping to the bus every morning for a 15-minute ride, and then waiting around for another bus to take me home sounded about as fun as the radiation itself. No way was this going to happen.

As we discussed the options, Dr. H mentioned that I could do radiation anywhere in DC—but that she wouldn't be able to be my doctor. In the short time I had been in Dr. H's office, I immediately liked her. She was warm, gentle and smart, and felt like someone I would have been friends with in another life. Needless to say, I was reluctant to work with another doctor.

When I told her that I lived a stone's throw from George Washington University Hospital, Dr. H suggested reasonably that I could meet with the radiation oncologist on staff there, if only to see whether I liked her. I sighed. Another appointment with another doctor felt like an ordeal. I was definitely experiencing appointment-fatigue at this point, unsure if I was even capable of meeting yet another doctor, especially one I might not like.

George Washington University Hospital is a teaching hospital so there are always a number of residents and interns poking and prodding during doctor appointments there. This was one of the reasons I was initially relieved to find out that my surgeons were associated with Sibley. Tucked away in the Palisades in upper Northwest DC, Sibley is quiet and a lot more private. But after learning that radiation is more of an in-and-out type of treatment, I wasn't so sure quiet and privacy mattered as much.

About a week later I found myself at the now-demolished Warwick Building, affiliated with but not attached to GW Hospital. There, I met with Dr. S, my second potential radiation oncologist in a week. As I walked into the pre-war style building on the corner of 23rd and K St., I looked around and immediately thought to myself, "This sure as hell ain't Sibley." Sure, it was convenient—a mere five minutes from my apartment (versus five miles away and only accessible by bus). But the walls and the floor were drab and dark and the waiting room seemed ancient in comparison to Sibley's fancy pants cancer wing.

Dr. S was fine. I definitely didn't get the warm fuzzies from her in the same way I had with Dr. H. But as I soon learned, I really wouldn't be seeing her all that often since the actual radiation is done by the technicians.

"You'll do," I said after meeting with her, checking "find radiation oncologist" off my list of things to do. I remember making my way back to my apartment tremendously fatigued, looking forward to taking a well-deserved nap. I was both physically and existentially tired, and in some ways was feeling simply defeated. When would this all end? When did my pulled muscle-turned cancer-turned mastectomy-turned chemotherapy-now turned radiation end? The answer isn't simple, because as much as they tell you that there is an end to it all, there isn't.

Radiation Station

Radiation is a process that will begin with a tour of the radiation facilities. Since getting radiated involves, well, actual radiation, most facilities will cloister off the treatment location. As a result, it seems like there is top secret testing going on in the basement, and that's where you will ultimately end up. I liked to think of it like Dr. Evil's underground lair because doing so in any other way would've made me too depressed.

The radiation center at GW is in a building that time apparently forgot. When I was a patient there, the waiting room was dark and dingy and adorned with really bad and dated magazines. To make up for it, there was free coffee and tea, which was a plus because I like free things, especially when I have to sit and wait. On my first visit, I wasn't there to radiate yet, just to meet with my new radiation oncologist, tour the facilities and to receive my first set of tattoos that help to ensure that the radiation technicians get the same spot each time, which in theory makes sense, but tattoos? The ins and outs of cancer and its treatment were getting more and more ridiculous.

I met with Dr. S and soon learned that it didn't really matter if I liked her or not because I would only be seeing her once a week for all of five minutes. The rest of the time I would be in the hands of the radiation technicians who happened to be super nice and knew exactly what they were doing. This was a huge relief because the last thing you want is an inexperienced person aiming radiation at your body.

After Dr. S and my discussion, she led me to the elevator, and instructed me to go down one floor to meet with the technicians who were waiting for me. As the elevator slowly creeped its way down to the depths of the building, I wondered what awaited me on the other end. Just then, the doors opened and a slender, youthful looking Ethiopian woman (who was no taller than 5'2) stood before me.

"Hello Ms. Goldberg. My name is E. I am going to be your radiation technician."

She was too cute for word so I had to say it: "What are you like 12? You're so young!" I exclaimed.

She laughed. "No, Ms. Goldberg. Please come with me and I will show you where to change."

I followed my new friend into what looked like a high school locker room and she pointed to a stack of gowns.

"You can put your things in the locker and undress from the waist up. The gown opens in the back and when you are finished, come outside and sit in the chairs outside the door."

I nodded and as soon as she left, took my shirt off for the zillionth time and donned yet another starchy robe with geometric shapes on it and I wondered who the designer was for this line? Can you imagine someone sitting in some room thinking, "what kind of design can I put on a hospital gown to make it look just appealing enough?"

With my floor-length gown, untied in the back, I sat in the hallway and waited for my new friend to come and get me. When she reappeared, she led me down the hallway to the radiation room which would be the control center for Dr. Evil's empire, had that been where I actually was.

The first thing that anyone notices about the radiation room (and how can you not) is the door. This is not any old door. This door is made out of industrial metal, and is about a foot wide and maybe six feet tall. It is machine operated and when it closes, it sounds like all of the air in the room is going to be sucked out and you are going to die.

Once the door closed behind me and E, I looked around the room. It was pretty bare bones, with the exception of this monstrous machine, of course. The machine sat menacingly in the middle of the room: a long, sliding table with a giant octopus arm dangling above it.

"Lay down on the table," E instructed. "We'll get your imaging set up and give you your tattoos so when we start radiation next week we'll know where you should be positioned every time you come in.

Dr. S had spoken to me about these tattoos and at first I was not super thrilled about it, not because I am against tattoos—quite the opposite, in fact. I've actually wanted a tattoo since my early 20s. Every trip I've ever taken to Las Vegas has always included a portion of the trip during which I would stare wistfully into a tattoo parlor, trying to decide what to get that I wouldn't regret. Thus far in my life, nothing had come to mind.

These tattoos were not going to be anything like what I had envisioned; first of all, they were not going to be administered by some artist-type, sleeved and pierced. These were going to be given to me by my new friend E and rather than a star or a bunch of letters or a catchy phrase in an array of colors, these were going to be dots. Blue dots. Yes, blue. Blue dots at various points on the left side of my body, since that was the side I was getting radiated. I do not know the reasoning behind why the dots (or their real name, markers) have to be blue; in fact, no one seems to because I asked around. But the dots had to be blue.

"Has no one ever asked this question?" I said to E as she prepared her small needle.

"Why has no one asked that?" I pressed. "I mean, permanent blue dots? Why can't they be black or brown so they look more like normal freckles rather than Smurf freckles?"

E shrugged and I gave up the conversation. Clearly she had no idea and I was just prolonging the inevitable.

I laid still as the room grew dark and lights were illuminating the left side of my body where E was making markers so she knew where to put the tattoos. There really is nothing worse than your tattoo artist giving you a Smurf dot where you don't need one, that's what I always say.

When she had the markers in place, she began her tattooing, which did not hurt at all, considering they literally were tiny blue dots; two on either side of my waist, one on either side of my left breast and then a few more around it, just for good measure. The entire process took no more than 15 minutes.

Once she was finished, E sat me up and handed me a cloth drenched in rubbing alcohol.

"You'll need this to get the marker off," she said. "You can go back into the changing room and get dressed and we'll see you back next week to start your radiation treatment.

Confused about the dripping cloth, I walked back to the changing room to get dressed, I looked in the mirror and that's when I saw it.

My body, unlike the title of John Mayer's sultry 2000s hit, had not become "a wonderland," but rather a treasure map. Black and blue marker had been drawn all over my chest with large X's where the tattoos now permanently lived on my body. I stared in the mirror in horror before beginning a massive scrub down, in that moment, understanding why this cloth was absurdly drenched. A good five minutes of scrubbing later, I emerged from the locker room, my chest still showing the faint hint of marker that was had just encompassed my entire body.

"Ok, Ms. Goldberg, we'll see you back here on Monday to start your radiation. Your time slot is 9:00am every day," E said as I waited for the elevator to take me back up to sea level.

"Works for me," I responded. I had wanted a time earlier in the morning so that I would have to wake up before 9:00am to keep my body on some sort of normal schedule so that when I did return to work my body would not go into shock. I also just wanted to get it out of the way earlier in the day rather than later.

With my tats in place and my radiation slot scheduled, I was allowed to take the rest of the week off so I could enjoy some time that did not involve radioactive waves, chemotherapy or any other doctor for that matter and went home to New York to see friends, visit with my parents and try to forget that treatment was by no means finished.

My six weeks of radiation felt like listening to song on repeat. The process was consistent, tedious and more familiar each time. From 8:27am until 9:30am each morning, my routine was exactly the same. I would wake up, get dressed, take my 10 vitamins, walk across Washington Circle over to the Warwick Building, banter with the radiation receptionist, drink a glass of ice cold water in the waiting room, check my email and call my mother. When the receptionist called my name, I would take the elevator to the depths of the building, change into a starchy robe, and sit in the hallway until E called me into the room with the iron door. Once I was on the table, my left breast was radiated for about 20 minutes at three or four different angles, all with my left arm held over my head. Then I'd hop off the table, the iron door would slowly creek open, I'd go back into the locker room and take off my starchy robe, get dressed and walk back across the circle. I would typically arrive back to my apartment by 9:30am, at which point I could then actually begin my day.

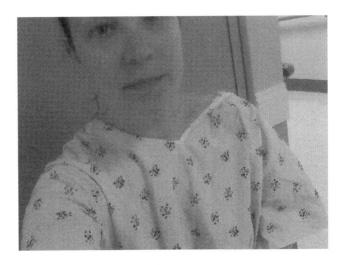

Radiation couture.

As predicted about half way through radiating, I began to notice that the left side of my chest was considerably darker than my right, and more specifically on the left side of my left breast, as well as in my left armpit and just below my armpit. "I'm getting so tan," I thought to myself. But the glow of radiation quickly turned into the bane of my existence five days later. Burns from radiation look and feel similar to regular old sunburns, but there's something that's just a little more intense about it. The feeling is more raw; the burn feels like it goes deeper than your run of the mill sunburn.

Dr. S had recommended a number of different lotions to soothe the burned areas of my skin. But what I had found that worked best was the prescription cream that I had asked my plastic surgeon to prescribe to me for the freezer burn that I had a tendency to get right where my hairline met my forehead from using the cold caps during chemotherapy. It was the one tricky spot where if I put the moleskin too high, I'd end up ripping off chunks of my hair and if I put it too low; the result would be a freezer burn. Biafine is a cream created to cure first and second degree burns and to protect the skin from scarring and worked perfectly for both freezer burn and radiation burn. I would lather the left side of my body with the glue-like cream at night, heat emitting from my skin like I had just spent the day on the beach. Every morning, I noticed that my skin was getting redder and redder, but the Biafine took the sting out. I would have been covered in this cream all day long but you cannot have any lotions, perfume or deodorant on when you go to radiate so this routine was relegated to the evenings only.

By week six of radiation, I was four days away from my 33rd birthday. While "excruciating pain" may seem like a melodramatic phrase, it didn't strike me that way during my radiation process. Every morning when I put a bra on was, for lack of a better word, kind of excruciating. I could feel the rawness of my skin at every point of contact. Luckily, I didn't have much to do those days. Sometimes, as soon as I was in the privacy of my own apartment, I'd tear off my bra and spend the day on the couch covered in Biafine.

My last day of radiation was June 12, 2011 and my last day felt similar to my last day of chemotherapy. Six weeks of going to the same place at the same time every day, you know everyone's name, you know where you're going and you see people who are just starting on this part of their journey and all you want to do is tell them, "it'll be okay" and "you'll get through this." But again, you know that they're not in a place to hear that, because you weren't so you say nothing and go on your merry little way.

I thanked everyone for being lovely and making this annoying task not as bad as it could have been. Then, I walked home, put my "radiation diploma" on the fridge, sat on my couch and felt a big question descend upon me.

"Now what?" I asked out loud.

Chapter 6: Nothing is Good For You (February 2011 – January 2012)

January 21, 2011
Subject: Three Oh, Is a Magic Number

Other than being half way through treatments, my big news is that I added a new member to my arsenal of doctors... I, Meredith Goldberg, the chain-smoking, vodka-drinking, bacon-loving friend you all know has gone...natural. I know. Take a moment to absorb this news. It's a shock.

Since I have a constant flow of toxic drugs running through my system, I was kind of annoyed taking more pills when I wasn't feeling well, so I found me a Natural Doctor. And she's not just any natural doctor. This woman has a wall of pills, potions and eye droppers filled with natural goodness. Too bad it's all legal. I now have my own personal stash of natural supplements to cure the 8,000,000 side effects from chemo. I got more pills than I ever had in college...I got pills to boost my white blood cell count, pills to help me sleep better, pills to prevent side effects I don't even HAVE yet! It may seem insane to you, and does to me, too. But so far, it's been effective ... so I ain't complaining.

For all intents and purposes, I will never preach to anyone about how to eat. To me, food is fun. Food is life. I remember places I've traveled from the food I've gotten to try all over the world. Octopus on a stick in Japan, crispy pig's ear in the Dominican Republic, handmade pasta in Italy. You get the idea. The intricacies of creating the perfect meal and the accompanying dessert make me smile. I love to bake. I love to create in the kitchen. My cobalt blue

Kitchen-Aid has since been with me in the front seat of every apartment move since 2003. It should be no surprise then that all the effects this process has had on my body, and particularly on my taste in food, were tough pills to swallow.

For someone who loves food, cancer, chemotherapy and everything afterwards is somewhat of a death-sentence for your palate. Not only are you probably going to be advised by doctors to shy away from foods that you love, but many patients find that food just doesn't taste the same after the first round of chemotherapy. For some, shifts like these are temporary; for others, taste buds never quite fully recover. Bland will take a new form of meaning and your ability to withstand spicy food will likely undergo a drastic recalculation. And of course, then there are the delicious foods that you are told plainly to stay away from during and after treatment: you know, like evil, refined sugar and any animal products.

For me, food and cancer options and theories and studies are like assholes: everyone's got one. What's the "best" way of eating? I have no idea. Will I forever spend my life searching for the answer while sucking down glass after glass of veggie juices? Probably not.

Have I learned what my body can digest and what it can't and what makes me feel better and what doesn't? Yes.

The bottom line is that everyone will have different reactions to different foods during this process. I can tell you what happened to me and how I dealt with it, and even how I would torture myself by watching Paula Deen at my lowest, queasiest point of my chemo treatment, clinging to the hope that some of her buttery goodness would come through the screen.

My Foodography

My story with food and my palate is like following a game of Candy Land. Starting at the no carb, all meat forest, through the salami and vodka foothills, down the organic trail and ending up somewhere in the middle of the board. I never wanted to be hyper-conscious of the foods that I put into my body.

In fact, I never really subscribed to the fad diet world until my senior year of college when Oprah did a show on people who were addicted to carbs. Chrys and I were still living together at the time. As we watched Oprah's special, we looked at each other with solemn recognition: "That's us! We're addicted to carbs!" And thus, the no-carb, Atkins revolution was born. All meat, all the time. We tossed the bread and lived on meat and cheese. Well, meat and cheese and cigarettes and vodka—I mean, it was college after all. I shunned carbs at all costs, including most fruits. I was a candidate for rickets, but I lost weight and managed to keep most of it off for a very long time.

My post college diet was pretty similar to college: meat, cheese, vodka, cigarettes. The only fruit that I "ate" was lime, which I squeezed into my vodka sodas. Sure, I could cook; I'd make the occasional turkey meatloaf with yummy ketchup and mustard topping, but desserts were my thing. I've always loved the precision of baking—how leveling the teaspoon of baking powder in a cake recipe would ensure a cake that was fluffy, moist and delicious. The baking gene was passed down from my grandmother. Her cookies and honey cakes were the talk of the Five Towns on Long Island growing up. You couldn't pay a Shiva call on Long Island or in Boca Raton without seeing it cut into perfect squares; hunks of moist cake, sweetened with creamed honey with toasted slivered almonds sprinkled on top, the corners slightly browned and protected by brown paper bags from Key Food. Grandma Ruth's baking was perfection and few in my family carry the baking gene. As we'd learn in time, the BRACA gene was another story.

As for my baking style, I'd make pineapple cheesecakes for luau-themed holiday parties, egg nog cheesecakes for Christmas, carrot cakes for Easter. But when it came to cooking for myself, I always made something easy. Throw together a few veggies; roast an entire squash—all things that were simple, fast and cheap. I always hated doing dishes and since in the 15 years I've lived in apartments around DC, exactly one of them has had an actual dishwasher. The more one-pot meals, the better.

When Washington, DC went into foodie mode, I went along. I was working in public relations at a hotel and loved spending time in the hotel's different kitchens. The fine dining chef was French and stereotypically nasty. The café chef was French and young and innovative and the hotel's Executive Chef was, well, just like every other hotel executive chef you've ever met. They are paid the most, think they're the best, cook really well, drink too much, smoke too much and don't generally stay in one place for very long. My local celebrities weren't politicians, they were chefs. I squealed when I saw Michel Richard sitting at the bar of his own Central and blushed the first time I saw Jose Andres. This was the world I loved; this was the world I wanted to know about.

By 2010, the year I was diagnosed, my love for food had reached a fever pitch, I had set up a Twitter account simply so I could follow all of the food trucks in DC, just in case I had a craving for a lobster roll, frozen yogurt or Korean BBQ at any time of the day. I wanted to try every restaurant, eat every animal and become a butcher. And then my taste buds were smacked with a harsh reality.

The first few days after my initial diagnosis, I went directly to my go-to comfort food: carbs and bacon. For many, comfort is something sweet. For me, it's bread, warm and chewy with butter. Second to my love of bread is my love of bacon. Crisp and greasy and delicious. As a Jew growing up on Long Island, one would think that bacon was not in my vocabulary, but this is 100% incorrect. Every summer, my parents and I would escape to the Catskills where my grandmother, a Florida snow bird, owned a small cottage that we would visit every summer. Once my grandmother had passed away, the house became ours and our first meal every time we arrived each summer? BLT sandwiches. I have very vivid food memories of unpacking my clothing and running down with my father to feel the temperature of the lake (which was always cold) as my mother would stand in our very 1970's tiny kitchen and crisp up about a pound of bacon that the three of us would finish in about 20 minutes.

These were (and still are) my favorites and my go-to's when something in my life has gone terribly wrong. Cancer warranted the mass consumption of both. Little did I know that these two items would become more of a luxury as my path to being "well" continued.

Nutrition as an Afterthought

I soon learned that battling cancer not only involves taking the drugs that have been created to cure the disease, but also making sure to monitor the food that you put in your mouth. That said, the second part is something that your doctors will never tell you. It's not because they are trying to keep you from being generally healthy and dependent upon synthetic medicine. The reason that they don't tell you this is because they don't know. Most oncologists, surgeons, and just about any other doctor that is specialized to help you cure your cancer don't have any training in nutrition, which was first brought to my attention in the 2008 film *Food Matters*. To be honest, I was kind of baffled by how little my doctor's knew about the importance of diet. Why wouldn't doctors want to understand the intricacies of food and how certain foods affect the body?

Regardless of the details, the final take away is this: your doctor isn't going to tell you how to go about exploring the best diet for your body, so it's up to you to make it a priority to learn about foods that will make you feel better and the supplements that can help keep you from getting sick (especially when going through chemotherapy, which will assault your immune system).

There is so much information out now about food and what's good for you and what isn't that it's often hard to separate what's fact from fiction. You'll come across books that tell you that eating animals and dairy will make you sick and then there are diets that are convinced that meat-based diet is most healthy. Despite how cancer has affected my body and understanding of nutrition, I still believe that food is an experience, and that you should enjoy every minute of it. So when reading the nutrition books you encounter or when doing your research online, remember that it's still important to keep your mind open to trying new foods, flavors, cooking techniques and point.

Case and point. During my carb-free days pasta was my enemy. I wouldn't even look its way at the grocery store. Rice? Forget about it! Sure, I'd order pounds of chicken and broccoli when getting Chinese food, but the small container of rice that came with it went right in the garbage. I could have fed a small army with the amount of rice I've discarded in the past. Somewhere in the mid 2000's when quinoa came onto the scene I was at a Pleasance's house for dinner and she had made it as a side dish.

I looked at it quizzically, "What is that?" I asked.

"It's quinoa. It's a grain. Try it."

I took a fork full and immediately fell in love. It was nutty and hearty and was slightly reminiscent of pasta. "This can't be good for you, it must be full of carbs," I thought to myself as I put my fork down.

"It's not like pasta." My friend shook her head at me, as she noticed me slowing down. It's a grain, not a simple carbohydrate."

Until this time, I never really fully understood the difference between simple and complex carbohydrates. And after being told that carbs were my enemy for so long, I just ignorantly avoided everything that resembled a carbohydrate, without taking into account this essential distinction. I had been programmed in such a way that I wouldn't touch anything that was high in carbs, even if it was also high in fiber or protein. But quinoa—a protein-rich grain– was eye opening to me. It meant that I could eat foods that kind of (at least to me) resembled pasta in a form that wouldn't affect me in the same way. Amazing. After this revelation, I started to amend the foods I ate. Slowly, I learned more about grains and whole wheat and complex carbohydrates rather than simple ones.

I tell you this story so you understand where I was coming from with food when I was diagnosed. Compared to people in the rest of this country who mostly consume highly processed foods (mainly due to the fact that they are a. cheap and b. readily accessible), I was a little further ahead in my foodography. But it was still a learning curve.

When most people think of chemotherapy, they have images of women sucking down ice pops in plush chairs. This is false. As I already said, the chairs are not usually plush, and secondly, ice pops are not always the best thing to be shoving into your mouth. If you've ever looked at the side of a box of popsicles, you'll see words like blue 1, red 40 and yellow 5. These are not football plays—these are actual ingredients! Now, maybe it's just me, but if you're already dealing with a slew of chemicals being pumped directly into your body, then why would you want to add more to the mix?

Enter the Alternates

Up until a few months into my diagnosis, my diet and overall lifestyle had changed in a way that seemed drastic to me. But compared to what I was then about to learn, the change was nothing. I wasn't really sure what I was supposed to be eating or avoiding, but the first decision I made was to buy exclusively organic fruits and vegetables. Since no one knew where my cancer had come from (and since we knew that it *wasn't* due to the BRACA gene), I wasn't going to take any chances with the food that was comforting me this entire time. Out went anything with an ingredient I couldn't pronounce, out went anything made with processed sugar and white flour. By the time I had purged my refrigerator, there was nothing left but mustard and a Brita.

What ensued was a series of substitutions. I replaced synthetic diet iced tea with Kombucha, which happens to be rich in probiotics, which are amazing for your body in terms of cleaning you out, keeping your energy up and warding off illnesses. My little pink packets of Sweet-n-Low were now white packets of Stevia, an all-natural, plant-based sweetener. My freezer, which used to be stocked with frozen veggies from Trader Joe's, was now empty, except for a bottle of Stoli and a pack of Marlboro Lights from Greece that I was saving for a special occasion. Yes, friends, I was a full on, BTS (big time smoker) before my diagnosis and this breakup was one of my saddest.

When you're diagnosed with a disease like cancer, some of your closest friends will not travel on with you. There will inevitably be a breakup—one that you saw coming for a while, but never wanted to let go of. No, I'm not talking about your 3am "friend with benefits." (But, for the time being you may want give that relationship a rest as well). I'm talking about you and your cigarettes. In my case, it was me and my Parliaments. We'd been together for about 15 years, give or take a year of Newport Lights and Marlboro Lights. 15 YEARS. We were committed to another, although in the last few months before I had gotten sick, we had definitely drifted save for our last ditch effort in Greece where we tried our hardest to stay together.

Once I had gotten back from my trip, Parliaments and I needed a little break from one another. Just as we were getting ready to make amends, I got sick and we had to say goodbye. I didn't really have a choice. It's like when you see a pregnant woman with a glass of wine at dinner, or out at a bar. Don't pretend like you don't judge her because you do. If anyone I knew saw me smoking they'd be like, "What the hell is she doing? She has cancer."

I had never tried to quit before, so I had no idea what it would be like. Would I crave cigarettes? Would I ever not carry them with me? These questions were easily answered over time. Don't get me wrong, there were times before my surgery when I would feel so defeated and angry and tired that I'd say fuck it and have one. But I better beat it to the punch, and surprisingly, it wasn't that difficult for me. To this day, the ease with which I quit smoking still baffles me. How could something that was so part of my daily routine become suddenly absent from my life?

A few months after I had my last cigarette, I was celebrating New Year's Eve and hadn't had a cigarette since August (we're looking at a six month hiatus). I was knee deep in the middle of chemotherapy and had two glasses of wine, which was a rarity for me during this time, and then I smelled my old friend coming from the porch. It was almost like it was calling out to me, "Meredith....we're heeeeeerrreeeee". I walked outside, as if in a trance, or more like Tucan Sam, following my nose and there was Ricky, smoking a cigarette.

"Give me a drag," I said, as if I hadn't skipped a beat.

He looked at me with that, "Do you really want to do that?" face and I gave him my, "don't lecture me" face. He reluctantly handed the Parliament over.

I took a drag and then it happened. That burning, aching feeling that a smoker gets when they try to smoke when they're sick with a nasty cold. Pain, discomfort and zero joy. I handed the cigarette back to Ricky and shook my head. My old friends had abandoned me: we'd been together for 15 years and now, I can't take one drag without feeling like crap. I sighed and went back inside.

To this day, I'll still perk up when I smell a cigarette from time to time. This is something that non-smokers will never really understand and I know, it's better that way. Smoking is a filthy habit and one that I loved from the minute Michelle and I bought our first pack of Virginia Slims when we were 15 and tried to light one on the windiest day of the year in a park by my house on Long Island. For almost a year after my diagnosis, I carried my last pack of Parliaments with my last cigarette with me at all times and when I would walk into one of my many doctor's offices and my bag was open, they'll give me the, what I like to call "The Doctor Eye."

Picture your doctor quickly tilting his or her head to the side with a raised eyebrow. This is The Doctor Eye. "I just carry them," I'd explain. They would half nod, half shake their heads in confusion. I'd shrug my shoulders.

Although I knew that quitting smoking was a no-brainer, I wasn't sure what changing the food I ate was going to actually do for me, but when you have a disease and you aren't sure where it came from or how to keep it at bay, you tend to be more open to try anything. It wasn't until speaking with nurse T to learn about the side effects of chemotherapy when I first began to see how the food you eat actually can change how you feel.

At my second meeting with nurse T, she supplied me with yet another packet of information that I really didn't want to read. On one sheet was a list of foods that I should eat the day of and after a treatment. White bread, Jell-O, pudding, chicken broth. Yuck. How could this be possible? How could Jell-O, a snack that has zero nutrients or health benefits be on a list of approved foods to help you feel better after being injected with toxic chemicals for hours on end? There was no mention of grains, fruits or vegetables. No. This could not be correct. I silently put the reading materials into my bag and began my own research.

One of the benefits of having cancer in a large city is that there are a plethora of alternative doctors and nurses and holistic wellness facilities that are begging you to seek alternative healing modalities. The day I was diagnosed, Pleasance began sending a steady stream of resources around Washington, DC regarding alternative medicine, acupuncture, yoga classes, natural products, you name it. While she had been disseminating this information to me for years, I'd always taken her suggestions with an, "Oh, that's cool" air. Yet, there I was, the same person who joked with her just months before getting sick that I would never stop using pore-clogging, aluminum-laden antiperspirants. "Maybe I'll get cancer, but at least I'll never smell," I'd tell myself. It wasn't until after my first chemotherapy treatment that I began actually understanding what alternative medicine was all about. I have to tell all the skeptics out there, what I learned saved me days on the couch, cleared up my skin and when the chemo. When radiation were both over, I realized that I had actually never felt better.

Taking the First Step

After extensive research and reading about alternatives that would make me feel better (since you know I had the time), I found myself making my first appointment with a Naturopath. What is a Naturopath you ask? As explained on my ND's website, "Naturopathic physicians are holistic primary care physicians. Naturopathic doctors diagnose and treat the full-spectrum of chronic and acute conditions. Because they address the whole person and seek out the cause of symptoms and conditions, naturopathic doctors offer an effective array of approaches and treatments for otherwise complicated health problems."

My parents, many of my friends and of course my oncologist thought I was insane, but I was excited to investigate this side of wellness, especially since I didn't have much else to do with my time. Why not explore something that could make me feel better rather than lying on the couch waiting to feel better?

I compare my first appointment with my ND like going to a new country. You don't speak the language. You aren't sure about what you're about to be eating, but you're almost convinced it's the best thing ever. As I walked into Dr. O's office, I was immediately intimidated by the floor to ceiling bottles of pills, herbs and eye droppers of remedies I couldn't pronounce. Her desk looked so small in comparison to the copious bottles that lined the walls, as did she. Dr. O was a younger woman with a mess of brown hair, and there was just something about her that put me at ease. You would think that after the barrage of doctors' visits to which I had already been subjected, this appointment would be a walk in the park, but it wasn't. For the first time, I was asked to describe in detail everything from how I was feeling emotionally, to the things I ate, plus every squeak or crack that my body. For the first time ever, really, I was being forced to take a minute to listen to what my body was telling me, and do nothing else. I know it may sound strange, but I also know that spending this time and energy to take full stock of my body was what allowed me to play a more active role in helping myself heal.

I've spent two hours waiting for a doctor before, but I had never spent two hours talking to one, and that's exactly what happened at my first appointment with Dr. O. My naturopath asked me to talk about what had been going on with me from the time of my diagnosis to the present, which was in December 2010. At this point, I was already one chemotherapy treatment in, and had already been sick for about three weeks and not just chemo sick, cold sick. It was the constant winter cold that brought me to make my first appointment. When they tell you about the side effects of chemo, they tell you about the nausea and the intense exhaustion. But no one tells you about how weak your immune system gets—how just walking past someone who has a cold could put you indoors for a week. In short, chemotherapy attacks everything in its path, meaning that it weakens your body

I had been sneezing up a storm since Thanksgiving and felt generally miserable. Dr. O explained to me that the chemotherapy was essentially fighting with everything in my body like a schoolyard bully. Some parts of my body were able to fight back, but others, like my white blood cells and the stomach enzymes meant to help me digest food, were like the short kids that always lost their lunch money. This is why I was left with what felt like a permanent cold and a weak stomach.

Dr. O explained some theories about cancer that stemmed from more alternative medicinal traditions. For instance, ancient Chinese medicine regarded cancer as an inflammatory disease. Today, inflammatory disease is described in the following, rather technical terms: "the inflammatory response directs immune system components to the site of injury or infection and is manifest by increased blood supply and vascular permeability which, in technical terms, allows chemotactic peptides, neutrophils, and mononuclear cells to leave the intravascular compartment. Microorganisms are engulfed by phagocytic cells (e.g., neutrophils and macrophages) in an attempt to contain the infection in a small-tissue space."[17] In other words, cancer, historically, was classified as a buildup within the cells, which makes them unable to perform properly. According to traditional Chinese medicine (TCM), this was often due to an imbalance in the body that could be balanced with herbs and food—not with chemotherapy, as we're apt to do in this day and age.

"It's no wonder you've had a cold for the past three weeks," Dr. O said as I blew my nose for what seemed like the tenth time that day, while she looked over my latest blood counts that she had asked me to bring.

"Here's what we're going to do," she continued, taking notes while she spoke. "We're going to go through each symptom you've been experiencing, and the side effects from the chemotherapy. From there, we'll figure out how to target each of those, and we'll use some preventative measures to keep you from getting sicker as you get deeper into your treatments."

"Sounds good to me," I replied, blowing my nose, again.

"Tell me what you've been eating," she asked.

Fast forward two hours: I walked out of Dr. O's office with a list of foods to eat and a list of what to stay away from, plus a routine of smoothies, vitamins and herbs all designated to prevent a different side effect of the chemotherapy and to make me feel better in general. The first was a new morning smoothie, the recipe of which was designed to awaken all parts of my body each day. One of the most central reasons for the smoothie was to have a vehicle to deliver myself Glutamine, a supplement that I was now supposed to be ingesting in pretty large quantities, especially given that the chemo was making it difficult for me to digest most foods. While most of what I was eating tasted like milky water or metal, I was still sometimes genuinely hungry. The problem was that whatever I put into my mouth then felt like it just sat in my stomach, unable to make its way through my digestive system. Simply feeding myself almost inevitably left me with a distended stomach and a bad attitude.

There were a few main supplements that I was instructed to take daily to prevent some of the side effects of the specific chemotherapy drugs from affecting my body. The first of these was the Glutamine, which comes in powder form and was incorporated into my morning smoothies along with frozen organic berries, a little almond milk and ground flax seeds. Flax seeds, as I learned over time, are not only amazing for your digestive system, but also act as a filter, absorbing toxins and helping your body get rid of them, almost like magical little sponges.

The Glutamine was not only designed to help with digestion, but was also to prevent neuropathy, a very common and evil side effect of chemotherapy. Neuropathy from chemotherapy typically affects the peripheral nervous system and it's symptoms tend to be: numbness, tingling (feeling of pins and needles) of hands and/or feet, burning of hands and/or feet, numbness around mouth, constipation, loss of sensation to touch, loss of positional sense (knowing where a body part is without looking), weakness and leg cramping or any pain in hands and/or feet or difficulty picking things up or buttoning clothes. The areas of the body most commonly affected are the extremities (hands and feet), but can really strike any part of the peripheral nervous system.[18]

The more Dr. O explained to me what this was, the more I realized that I did not want this to happen to me. As much as I couldn't always stomach the Glutamine, I drank my smoothie every morning and dutifully took two B6 vitamins and one Alpha-Lipoic Acid pill every morning without fail.

Next up was my battle with my white blood cell count. I had already been relegated to two Nupogen shots after each round of chemo and still my white counts were only at a 1.0, when normally they should be around 8.0. For this, I was taking six immune-building supplements per day, which were all made solely out of different mushrooms. Two times a day, I would put 10 drops of Medulloseinum Plex into whatever it was I was drinking, which was usually either green tea or water. Unfortunately, the more chemo treatments I had, the worse water tasted, so for the most part it was green tea. Medulosseinum Plex is a homeopathic product specifically formulated to reduce the effects of trauma to the skeletal system and to enhance the healing of bone, tendon, periosteum and ligament injuries, so basically, it was trying to naturally do what the Nupogen was doing, repair the bone marrow to produce more white blood cells.

The hardest thing to combat, and in some ways still is today, was my digestion. As I had said, food may have gone down, but it wasn't exactly ever ready to come out. When I did eat, I'd just feel the food collecting and sitting in my stomach, leaving me bloated and insanely uncomfortable. For this, Dr. O first started with my morning smoothie, digestive teas, probiotics and a radical change to my diet which from that point on, changed the way I ate for life.

"I'm going to ask you to try an anti-inflammatory diet during your treatment," Dr. O said.

"What's that?" I asked, curious.

As she explained, the basis of an anti-inflammatory diet is pretty simple. No gluten, very little meat (and if you're going to eat meat, it has to be grass-fed, antibiotic-free), no dairy or refined sugar. Gone were the whole grains I thought were helping such as wheat, spelt, barley, rye and kamut. Gone were the organic cereals that had still tasted normal as they were made wheat, as well as nightshade fruits and vegetables, which included potatoes, tomatoes, eggplant, bell peppers. Peanut butter was to be replaced with other nut or seed butters. Corn was out, as was anything made with corn products. Citrus was off the table, as was any fruit juice, dried fruit and alcohol. My head was swimming with questions. What the hell I was going to eat every day if all of these items were making my stomach worse? I thought I was already on the right track, having made with switch to all organic, but clearly, I had much to learn in the ways of nutrition. That was fine with me; I had the time to learn.

So, if you're keeping tabs, while most things on the shelves contain gluten, even more things contain corn. I can't tell you how many times I found myself standing in Whole Foods, exhausted from chemo, reading label after label, searching for something to eat. My relationship with my Anti-Inflammatory diet was not off to an easy start. Like a new boyfriend, every time I thought we were making progress, we'd take a step back. For ever cup of millet that I successfully cooked, I failed at properly cooking beans or legumes, not having soaked them long enough, leaving me with a pot of crunchy, tasteless lentils. Sometimes, I just went to bed angry and hungry. What did this mean for all the yummy dinners I wanted to try in my lifetime? What did this mean for my half-price bottle wine nights at my favorite local wine bar with locally-cured meats and cheeses?

Once the Anti-Inflammatory diet and I got into our groove, our relationship was a lot stronger and just like a good friend, I grew to depend on the diet to make me feel better. Armed with my list of foods and my tote bag, I scoured the famers markets in DC to find veggies and fruits that would keep my mouth happy even when everything tasted bland and metallic, rather than sucking down Jell-O like the instructions I had gotten from my oncologist. I learned to eat with the DC seasons (apples, pears and squashes in the fall and winter; asparagus in the spring; berries and zucchini all summer) and incorporating different types of beans into meals for added protein, resulting in an ongoing love affair with the chickpea (canned, I should say). The raw bean and I never made a great connection; I would never soak them long enough, never cook them long enough and never season them properly.

As I remained on this new path of eating, I started noticing changes to my body and how I felt overall. Little blackheads that I would get on occasion on my face? Gone. My hair and nails were growing at what felt like an exponential rate, which was certainly a plus since the chemo had left my nails pretty brittle. In general, I knew that I should be feeling a lot worse than I was and I think a lot of that was attributed to my diet and the supplements that I was taking.

I kept this regimen consistent through my chemotherapy and then continued with it through six weeks of radiation. Then, when it was all said and done, I figured, "Why stop now?" While I was done with chemotherapy and radiation, the toxins had pulled a number on my digestive system, leaving me still unable to digest white flour, processed sugars and certain raw vegetables like tomatoes and eggplant (both highly inflammatory foods). It was almost like my body was telling me that it had been through enough and appreciated this change in food and wanted it to stay that way, so who was I to argue? Which brings me to today, just about 5 years out of chemo and radiation. I don't even remember what I used to keep in my refrigerator before making the move to an anti-inflammatory diet. Don't get me wrong, I'll never say no to a dozen oysters, a bagel in New York or a night out with multiple dirty martinis. But when it comes to the question of how to make myself feel better, I've now learned to listen to what my body is telling me, whether it's saying that it's had too much or not enough of something. As a result, we've never been closer.

My naturopath has become a part of my forever-wellness team and was instrumental in helping my body readjust to working full time, which I'd been insanely nervous about for a number of reasons. Would my brain be able to keep up and better yet, would my body? I hadn't worked full time since the fall of 2010, so when I finally rejoined the work force in April 2012, I was worried about my stamina. And lo and behold, after my first week in the office, I got a cold. My body was not used to sitting in an office surrounded by other people, sans windows, for eight hours a day. My body missed natural sunlight, space and time to rest. I knew it was time to revisit Dr. O.

She quickly assured me that I, like so many others before me, was facing the same worries. What if it was stress that made me sick the first time? How do I prevent that going forward? How do I ensure that I'm being kind enough to my body so I can resume a normal life and keep myself healthy at the same time? The answer was fairly simple. Balance. It's all about keeping a balanced lifestyle that allows your body to rest yet push it in order to get yourself back into the swing of things.

The first thing Dr. O did was change up all of the supplements that I had been taking. Vitamin D was still a necessity as was a complex vitamin B. I had been taking Coq10 to help protect my heart during radiation since I was being radiated on the left side of my chest, but now that I was a year out from that, Coq10 was to be replaced with Fish Oil. Two anti-cancer supplements also entered my regimen: a complex immune/anti-cancer mixture of mushrooms and curcumin, the principal curcuminoid of the popular Indian spice turmeric, which is a member of the ginger family. I learned that curcumin was a potent anti-cancer supplement. I also learned that when a gel cap of curcumin opens by accident, it stains everything.

Armed with my new list of supplements, I felt more confident jumping back into working full time, but the question of food still remained. While I was "funemployed," I was eating at home all the time, which meant that I knew where my food was coming from at all times. Since I no longer had the luxury of eating at home, what was I to do? The answer seemed pretty simple: bag it.

My first few days of work I was taken to lunch by a few different managers and while everyone would order a sandwich from either restaurant in the hotel I was working at, I'd just get a salad and silently be very thankful that the main restaurant on my property was farm-to-table so I knew that everything I was putting in my mouth, I had likely seen at the same farmer's market that I shopped at every Sunday.

"You're being so good," my new coworkers would say after I'd ordered. I'd just shrug and smile, unsure how to answer that just yet, ruling out, "I can't digest most food from the intense six months of chemotherapy I went through,"

Once the welcome lunches ended and I had started making some work friends to have lunch with, we'd go downstairs to the employee cafeteria. If you've ever worked in hospitality, you know that it's like sleeping in steerage on the Titanic. While three floors above you guests are dining on farm-fresh salads and free range chickens, you are faced with defrosted vegetables and some kind of pasta smothered in various sauces throughout the week and hot dogs. No, this was not going to work for me, so I started bagging my lunch which mainly consisted of raw fruit and veggies.

"That's what you're going to eat?" "Isn't that boring?" "Why do you eat that every day?" These were just a few of the questions that I was faced with during my first few weeks back at the office—that is, until I was comfortable enough to share my story without getting "the look." And honesty, my new co-workers were so nice that I was a total non-issue once I just told the truth, but it definitely took a while. Now no one blinks when I walk into the office with a giant green juice or asks what diet I'm on when I decline the cake or cookies that are always around. And I don't always say no. I'll never miss an opportunity to get out of the office and gossip with my co-workers just because they aren't going somewhere organic for lunch. I refuse to be one of those people that brings their own food to another restaurant. That's just wrong.

Dr. O and I talked at length about this and how in these cases, the 80/20 rule will suffice. 80 percent of the time, I'm true to my anti-inflammatory diet and making sure that I'm doing something active with my body at least 3 times a week. The other 20? That's saved for nights out, enjoying the fact that I get a 20 percent. And that makes every bite of gluten taste that much better.

Chapter 7: So, What's Next? (June 2011 – Today)

June 12, 2011

A lot of people have told me how easy I make cancer sound in these funny, sardonic email updates. But the truth of the matter is, I would never have been able to go through all of this if I didn't have people that cared about me. I would have spent the last year curled up in a ball on the couch watching hours of bad cop shows (which I am now kind of addicted to) and wondering what the hell I was going to do with the rest of my life.

Now, don't get me wrong. I sometimes still feel sorry for myself and have "Why me?!" moments at least once a week. But all the time? Nope, that's just not how I wanted this all to go down, and I'm pretty happy with the way it turned out. Sure...I had cancer. And sure, I'll have this experience floating over my head for the rest of my life. But I get the rest of my life to handle it, and to me, that's kind of the best part of it all. Plus, I get to annoy the hell out of ALL OF YOU forever, and for that, I feel pretty lucky. I don't know how you all feel about it—but honestly, I don't care. you're stuck with me.

So here you are. Your chemotherapy has been completed, your radiation is done, your MRI's have come back clean. And while you still might have your *Holy-shit-I-am-exhausted* days, you're feeling OK for the most part. Now what?

For some, being sick is the easy part: you know what's coming, you know the routine. After the first round of chemo, you have a pretty good idea of how you're going to feel each subsequent time. After radiation, you know how what's going to happen to your body. But what happens once all of these wonderful steps towards recovery are over and you've been given the go-ahead to resume your "normal" life?

Well, no one really tells you that this step might be the most difficult, or at least no one told that to me. So that's why I'm telling you: this part is tricky. Your doctors might make it seem so easy, but it's not. On my first Herceptin-only treatment, I was meeting with my oncologist when he said to me, "It's time for you to rejoin the world." *Rejoin the world???* I thought to myself. I thought I'd been in the world-ish for the most part. I'd been going out, I made plans with people, I had a semi-job. But the reality was that I had been living almost a half-life, at least compared to my previous lifestyle. I had made so many huge changes in the year that I was sick and in treatment. I had pretty much abandoned my Bacchanalian existence for a more quiet and introverted way of life, which involved a lot more solo evenings in my apartment than out. And because the bulk of my treatment had ended in June of 2011, I felt almost like a kid with the summer off. I knew I had to find myself a job and try to figure out how to live a more balanced and less hermetic lifestyle. But I never really stopped to think about how that would happen, and how hard it would be to just jump back into a life that had totally evolved since August 2010. During my post-treatment phase, I found myself at almost my lowest point. I was, as I like to put it, "falling off the rails."

On the surface, I was "fine, just bored." I needed to keep busy, so I buried my head in doing things like writing, keeping cool (literally: I hate the summer) and just hanging out with friends once they were done with work each day. I spent a week in the Catskills with my parents in our tiny bungalow with no TV, no internet and no cell service. Most of that week was spent lying on the dock by the lake, looking up at the clouds and wondering, "What the hell am I doing?" I hadn't expected to still be looking for gainful employment; the effects of the economic shit show were unfamiliar to me. I thought for sure I was owed something great in return for the year that was just taken from me. This brings me to an interesting issue that I'm sure many people recovering from long-term illnesses also have pondered—the question of what you are owed.

After recovery, there seems to be this lull in one's life where you are waiting for something to happen. You've been through the icky parts, and now you expect there to be some light at the end of the tunnel. You might even expect something great to happen, or perhaps more accurately, you believe you are owed something. You've just spent a year, or however long, fighting to be well, fighting to be alive. Where's the payoff?! As Pleasance had put it, a difficult experience like pregnancy at least gives you a person in the end. But with cancer, there's no parting gift—you don't get to take anything home. Cancer is like a full-time job insofar as you have a place to be and something to do all the time. So as a result, many of us believe that we deserve compensation of some kind, something other than just getting better. But that doesn't just happen. For me, at least, the aftermath of surviving cancer was way harder than I had imagined.

Admittedly, I was expecting things to just fall back into place without any hard work of my own. I had just spent the past year doing all of the heavy lifting, and wanted a break. My body endured the surgery, the chemotherapy, the radiation, the physical therapy. I believed that the universe should've handled the rest, although that sounds naïve to say. Why should looking for a job or getting a piece published in a magazine be so difficult? Why should dating again be so laborious? Shouldn't these things just happen and work out for me? Didn't I deserve things to simply fall back into place?

As I pondered these questions while wandering the streets of DC one afternoon in December 2011, it hit me. I must've been somewhere between Foggy Bottom and Georgetown on one of my aimless day walks, and the light-bulb went off: I got to live. That was my reward. "Oh," I said out loud. "I am alive."

I'm not saying that this is an easy revelation to have. And once you're there, it's still kind of a challenging concept to grasp, especially when you're young. In your 20s and 30s it's kind of a given that you get to live, and to live well. You get to fall in love; you may get married and get to have children. But in some cases, this doesn't happen for you when it happens for everyone else. While you've been fighting simply to see your 35th or 40th birthday, everyone around you has gone about their lives. They've gotten engaged, married, and in some cases, even divorced. They may be starting or expanding their family, getting promoted or starting new jobs, and then there's you: you're on the outside looking in, and it's undoubtedly difficult. Often times, I felt like I was not a part of this exclusive, normal life progress club that seemingly everyone got to be a part of. Of course, I will forever be part of a totally different club. I may not know what it's like to walk down the aisle yet, but I do know what it's like to fight for the chance to put that dress on. No, that doesn't make it any easier—but you catch my drift.

Living in DC with an amazing group of friends who all happened to be married and/or starting their families was really difficult for a while. I often felt resentful of them and often became bored when we hung out. I was ready to live, but everyone had already been living and was settling down. I felt like a kid on Christmas who just wanted to run downstairs and open all the presents at 5:00am while my parents were still in bed, shooing me away. This stung because I love my friends, and I certainly didn't want to go out and make new ones. But something had to give if I was going to be able to stay in DC. Either I had to come to terms with what was happening around me, or I had to pack it up and start fresh somewhere else, which at the time, was New York City. I know NYC, I have friends (read: single friends) in NYC, I have family in NYC. I knew I could uproot my life and relocate, though the thought of destabilizing my daily existence again so soon after the cancer seemed like too much of an undertaking. So I made the simple choice to stay where I was, and to work just a little bit harder to claim my place in the early 30s set of DC. Though up until April 2012, I had no idea what that meant.

Working

Many people have no choice but to work through their diagnosis and subsequent treatment. If you are one of those people, I give you an insane amount of credit. The day I found out what I was about to endure for the next year, I mentally checked out of anything that wasn't family, friend or health related. Needless to say, my first conversation with my new employer was interesting ... to say the least. She had been out of the office on my first day of work, leaving me alone in a cubicle with a laptop, the employee handbook and no idea what I was doing. (Plus, there was the fact that I had been ignoring around 500 phone calls from parents, friends and doctors since I was trying to give off the vibe that nothing was wrong.) When my boss returned to the office on my second day, she called me in to touch base. She had no idea what was coming next and frankly, neither did I. This was the first conversation that I was having about my cancer that wasn't with a friend or family member and I had no idea how it was going to sound coming out of my mouth to a stranger.

"How did your first day go," she asked as I sat across from her in her office?

"It was good. Everyone seems great." I paused. "I need to tell you something."

"Is this about why you had to push back your start date?" she asked.

"Yes. You aren't going to believe this, but I have breast cancer," I said, half laughing, half tearing.

The ironic part of it all was that I was assigned to head up my boss' pet project, a health and wellness group that she had begun working with when she had been diagnosed with breast cancer a year earlier.

She grew teary and apologized.

"I'm so sorry you have to go through this. I went through this. You'll get through it. It won't be fun, but you'll do it."

"I know I will. I just feel so bad that I'm doing this to you." This was an honest answer. I really did feel a level of guilt for letting her down. There was no way that I was going to be able to run accounts and be a publicist. I knew it and she knew it.

"Let me figure out what we're going to do and we'll talk tomorrow," she said.

"I haven't told anyone in the office," I said.

"Legally, I can't," she said. "But I am going to have to talk to my CFO about it."

"That's fine," I replied.

As I walked out of my boss' office, it occurred to me that I didn't have much of a vocabulary when it came to the notion of what was legal and what wasn't. It had crossed my mind, but I was in no place to actually formulate what these legal issues meant for me. I was more concerned at the time with getting my surgery scheduled and choosing what my new breast was going to look like than what I was going to do about work. Many of you will put work first, and in some ways I wish I had. Why? Because I wouldn't have found myself at the other end of the cancer spectrum: unemployed.

This is where I encourage you to check out the Cancer Legal Resource Center, an organization I didn't even know existed until after I was done with all of my treatments. They are a non-profit and will listen to your case for free over the phone if you feel like your rights in the workplace have been violated in any way before or after your diagnosis.[19]

At this point in time, I had no idea what the hell was going on or what was next for me. I knew that in three weeks from the day I had started at my new company I was slated to have my surgery and then six weeks after that and I had healed, I was going to start chemotherapy. But other than that, I had no clue. I'm not going to lie to all of you and tell you that I haven't been extremely lucky in the fact that my family was 100% financially supportive of me and whatever I was going to have to do next, whatever that entailed. But I knew one thing for sure, there was no way in hell that I was going to be able to be an Account Executive and a Publicist like I had been hired to do. It just didn't seem important and obviously I didn't have the headspace to work as well as I could.

Since I work in the world of marketing, something that can be done from pretty much anywhere in the world, the idea of remote working was not impossible. My boss and I decided that I would be kept on as a consultant, and that when I was ready to come back to the office "there would be something for me." These, my friends, are famous last words. Since I'd been working full time since the age of 21, I like to think that I've learned a few things in business. One: never trust anyone you work with since, for the most part, the office still remains a prime example of Darwin's survival of the fittest in its most civilized form. But stupidly, I believed my boss' words that there would be something for me when I was on the other side of my treatment. Oof.

No, I'm not going to tell you to trust or not to trust your boss since every job is different and we all have our own relationships with our bosses (or maybe you are your own boss, which is even better). But I will say this: GET. IT. IN. WRITING. All of it. Any conversation that you have with your boss if/when you decide how you are going to weather the cancer storm in your office must be documented. You may not know what's ahead of you, but you can ensure that you know what you are coming back to as long as you take the proper steps on the front end. You may not want to deal with it at the time since work will become secondary in your life for at least a little while, but putting those measures into place now will take the edge off when you are ready to ease back into the working world full steam ahead.

Let my story be a cautionary tale for the rest of you. When I was ready to come back to work, there was no work for me to do, which I found odd since my company was acquiring new clients at an alarming rate. As I emailed back and forth with my boss to try to find a place to "put" me, I was continually brushed aside. We repeatedly set up times to sit down and talk, but a day before each of those meetings, my boss would cancel. I was left dangling somewhere between semi-employed and totally fucked. While I was still working on projects for them during my renegotiations (including one rather large project with a very short turnaround time), no one was really giving me the time of day. I'd communicated with the team directly when I (gladly) accepted the project (since I was really not in a position to say no or turn down the hours), yet on the day I turned over the work to the project manager, I was left in the lurch. I had asked for feedback and never heard another word about it, despite my two subsequent emails asking if the client had liked the deliverables. In fact, the only way I knew that the client liked the work was a few weeks later when I clicked on their website to see *all* of my words on their site.

After constant emailing back and forth with my then-boss, I finally encountered the truth. It turned out that they had decided they were going to do all of their writing in-house, meaning there just wasn't a place for me there anymore. To be honest, I didn't want to go back there. My boss was running a disorganized ship that had been taking on project after project. During the time in which I'd been hired, repositioned and going through treatment, they had gone through three project managers and a handful of other staff members. The work environment seemed disorganized, to say the least. And as many of you will realize, you probably won't want to jump back into a life of chaos after undergoing such personal upheaval. Some of you may, since there are always people who are energized by the everyday hustle. But I am not one of those people. Yes, I wanted to get back into a routine, but I wasn't terribly seduced by the idea of working 10 hour days, and to climb a corporate ladder that I wasn't even sure I wanted to be on anymore. This was an odd realization for me.

After the news that my time as a consultant was essentially coming to an end, there really was only one option for me. Unemployment. My memories of unemployment stem back to when I was a kid and my mother was in-between one of her million jobs and when I was on vacation from school I would have to go with her to the unemployment office on Long Island and stand in a line that snaked around the entire office.

"Did you work this week?"

"Nope."

"Did you look for work?"

"Yep."

And that was it. Living in DC, where a vast majority of the population is on some kind of government assistance, I wasn't expecting much from the system other than a lot of red tape and waiting around for a check. I heard various stories about unemployment (or "funemployment" as I like to call it, since it makes it sound better than it really is). One person told me that they got their money from DC right away and never had an issue, while I heard other tales of people who had to go down to the unemployment office and learn about how to effectively search for a job, a task that sounded daunting and pointless, but typical for DC. Luckily, for me, applying for unemployment was fairly easy and done completely online.

So I was now in the system, and I had no idea what to do with myself. Finishing this book was my goal. But after a year of dealing with a pretty intense situation (both physically and emotionally), I often didn't feel like writing about it all day long. I'd sit and stare at my laptop trying to think of witty nuggets of advice to dole out, but nothing would come through my fingertips. I walked around DC a lot. I hung out with Pleasance and Saylor a lot.

I tried to keep some semblance of a schedule so that when I was once again employed my system wouldn't be shocked to the core. Up at 8:15ish every morning. No TV-watching until 5:00pm. Each day as filled as possible. This all worked for a little while, until I realized in the summer of 2011 that the job market was not in the same shape as it had been in September 2010.

DC residents like to joke that Washington DC is a bubble so events that affect the rest of the world tend not to affect the district.. In other words, there were lots and lots of boring (to me) association and government jobs. I had made a promise to myself: once I was better, I was only going to apply to jobs that appealed to me, jobs that I would enjoy. Since I had quite happily worked in hospitality earlier on in my career, I looked to get back into it, though found that it wasn't as easy the second time around. I'm sure it didn't help that I had been out of the hospitality world for about four years while I was collecting what I thought would be valuable experience as a marketing and account manager in the slower paced manufacturing industry. I wrote newsletters for HVAC units, articles for generators and press releases for bath fans, which is, admittedly, about as exciting as it sounds. As I wrote all this soul-crushing copy, I would stare out of my office window, overlooking the Georgetown waterfront and dream. "If I could do anything else right now," I'd think, "What would I be doing?" Those were the jobs that I was trying to find, and I found out the truth the hard way: those were the jobs that were, in 2011, impossible to get.

The jobs bubble had reached DC and my "Oh, it'll be so easy to find a job" attitude soon turned a bit sour. It went something more like this: "Shit. This is a lot harder than I thought it was going to be."

The market had changed drastically in a year. Jobs I could've been guaranteed a year ago were now just out of my grasp, with those with more experience back in the market. Interviews that typically would have been with one team member became 30 minute Powerpoint presentations with rapid fire questioning from ten team members and an eventual email saying that it had come down to me and one other person and that other person just happened to have a few more years of experience than I had.

This would bring anyone down and it did bring me down for a while. But you know what made it worse? The recruiters who told me to "keep my head up" and "stay positive." They were the people I wanted to kick in the face after each rejection. What did they know about staying positive? They didn't just go through what I had been through, and they still had a job! I remember in the spring of 2012, I was chatting with a recruiter. I was closing in on one year looking for a full time job, a traumatic experience that I was trying to explain to the recruiter.

"We've all been there before," she responded.

"You have a job. So no, you haven't been here before," I barked back.

I'm not proud that I snapped at this recruiter, and generally agree that it's important to stay positive and focus on the big picture in times of difficulty. But I also think it is totally acceptable to have days where you feel like shit and want to tell people being fake that they can shove their "positive attitude."

Nine months after I had officially severed ties with my previous company, I found a new job. Nine months. I had gotten to that point where my brain was slowly becoming a shadow of its former self. I wasn't sure what I was going to do, but I knew that if something didn't pop for me soon, there was going to be trouble. I knew that I could not spend another summer lying listlessly on the dock in the Catskills wondering what the hell I was going to do. I needed to be back in the real world. I needed to be busy. Between June 2011 and April 2012 I interviewed for about 15 different jobs, some of which I really wanted, some of which I really didn't. But in all cases, I went on the interviews regardless of personal feeling or dramatic expectations. I was simply looking for a place where I could just be a part of and ease back into the life I should have been living for the past year. The more I interviewed at different marketing communications firms, the more it became apparent to me that I wanted to leave that world and go back to hospitality. Armed with this realization, I focused on job listings in hospitality and felt much more empowered than I had when my search was sprawling and unfocused. Although I was able to remember just how crazy my time was during my first stint in DC hospitality, I also remembered how much I enjoyed being part of a 24-hour machine. Maybe it wasn't the best place for me with regard to my physical health. But for my mind, I needed the pulse. I knew that it was where I wanted to be.

I'm a believer in fate—being in the right place at the right time and meeting the right people when you are supposed to. I think that's what happened with me and my first job post-cancer at a smaller boutique hotel in downtown DC. I got the call about my new job on Friday, April 13th, which will now forever be a lucky day for me. There I was, wandering the streets, running errands for friends who had jobs when the HR department called and offered me the job. I accepted on the spot. I didn't negotiate, I didn't ask any questions, I just said "Yes, I'll take it," hung up the phone, called my parents and started to cry.

I took two weeks after the day I had accepted my new position to retrain my body so that it was prepared to work a normal

9-5 job (or in this case, an 8:30-5:30 job). I hadn't been in an office since the summer of 2010, which was nearly two years ago at this point. During those two weeks, I started waking up daily at 7:00am, taking morning test walks to my new office in order to see how long it would take to get there every morning. (The average, I found, was 20 minutes, give or take.)

I tore my closet apart and dug out the suits that had been sitting on hangers for the past two years. I then walked across the street to my dry cleaner, a small Asian woman who I had been bringing my clothes to for years, though who I hadn't seen during my two year job hiatus. (Plus: I had no need for her to dry clean the t-shirts and jeans that had been my uniform.)

"You get a job," she asked, as she counted the pants and suit jackets?

"Yep."

"This makes me so happy! For so long I see you walking back and forth, back and forth down the street with no place to go. I was worried about you."

I think she was just happy to get my business back, but I thanked her for her enthusiasm and continued to prepare myself for my re-emergence into the "real world."

My first day back in the office was surreal. I wasn't exactly nervous since it was a job I had done before (working in PR and marketing at a hotel), so the landscape was pretty much the same. Sure, the players had changed and the market was considerably different that my last hotel job, which was in 2005 when the hospitality world was a little more carefree. But all, in all, things were not that different.

There was an eerie calm that came over me as I walked into the door on my first day. I wasn't scared. This is just a job. It can't be that hard. Cancer is hard. Fighting exhaustion and nausea and dealing with numerous doctors all of the time is hard. This is a job. It will be more annoying than difficult. But there I was, sitting at my new cube, watching my Outlook rapidly fill up with emails from people who I had never met.

I still felt that I had a lot to prove, not only to my new employers, but to myself; I had been out of the game for two years. I still had a nagging case of chemo brain, meaning my thoughts were not always the most eloquent when they came out of my mouth. Yet my mind was ready to be busy again. It was ready to be challenged, ready to bring ideas to the table, ready for a seat at the big kid's table. I was right where I was supposed to be, mentally.

Physically, however, my body was in shock after day one. It was almost as if it were confused, and unsure of what I was doing to it. "Wait, why aren't we going for a run this morning? Why are we sitting all day? Who are all of these other people in the room? Where's the sun? Where are our sneakers?"

I got a cold after three days in the office. Three days. That was all it took for my body to reject working full time. I wasn't used to forced air and sharing an office with ten other people, but this was my life now and my body had to fall in line. I spent that first weekend on the couch, re-grouping and filling my body with vitamins and Kombucha, anything to boost my immune system. With this job, working from home was not an option.

Eventually, I found my routine, working the balance that I had talked with Dr. O about. I made sure that if I worked from 8am – 8pm one day, I would be sure to leave at 5pm the next day and make time to go for a run. If I worked over the weekend, something that often happens in both hospitality and public relations, then I made sure to take it easy the next week.

The same held true for my stress levels at work. If I made a mistake, rather than getting mad at myself and defensive toward others (as I had in the past), I accepted it and moved on. I did and still try to do my best to make sure that I'm never running around with my head on fire because there's a hotel emergency. This isn't brain surgery, no one will die if I post something on Facebook and it's spelled wrong. My motto that I often express to my co-workers, even today is, "Relax, no one's died; it's not like we're curing cancer in here." They laugh nervously, but it's true. To me, nothing will ever be as important as trying to remain as calm as possible at all times. And don't get me wrong, we all have our days where we want to maim a client or a co-worker for being annoying, but then that moment eventually passes and it's just not a big deal anymore.

Working in PR can breed anxiety and stress. I can remember my first PR job at another hotel in DC and when a writer was on deadline I'd have an internal panic attack about getting them the information on time. I'd wait anxiously for the chefs to send me recipes or for the General Manager to send me a statement. Not anymore. I didn't and still don't wait for it, I just do it. I used to wait for explicit instruction and direction but now, I just move full steam ahead until someone tells me to stop. It makes the day go by much faster than constantly hitting refresh on Outlook, waiting for someone to tell me what to do or approve my suggestion. Some people will say this kind of self-possession comes with age, and maybe that's true to an extent. Or maybe it's just that I've realized along the way that work isn't all there is in life. Now that brings me to play time…

Playing

Dating is hard no matter how many ways you look at it. Add to the mix the stress of having just gone through an illness—that doesn't make it any easier. Of course, I wasn't in a rush to get back out there; part of me was still regrouping from the end of my last relationship, which I never really had a chance to properly recover from. Note: by "properly recover," I mean that I didn't have enough time to make my fair share of stupid dating mistakes and have lots of one night stands. My relationship ended in February 2010 and I was diagnosed in August 2010 so there really wasn't a lot of "me" time before cancer took over my datebook.

Once I was done radiating in June 2011, part of me knew that I should start getting out there, I should be dating again, and in a half attempt, I joined a dating website, but would delete most messages for any would-be suitors. I just wasn't into it. As much as I wanted to be, I found it hard to take it seriously. Dating, as many of us know, is kind of like looking for a job. You need to be persistent, you need to be open to rejection and you need to willing to look outside of your comfort zone, since some of the best jobs and partners are lurking where you'd never expect them to be. But at that point, I was not only trying to recuperate my energy, but also couldn't take anything seriously. On top of that, my feelings on dating and marriage and the whole "happily ever after" myth had shifted dramatically.

I was and will probably be a romantic first and foremost. I love the idea of love, don't get me wrong, but there's something about a failed attempt at marriage that makes you stop and revisit the practicality of it all. Why does one HAVE to get married? Why do you HAVE to have children? I had spent so much of my teen years and early 20s fixated on my search for this great love that somewhere along the lines I think I had forgotten to love myself first and that's a lot of what I learned with my therapist, Dr. G. Will I ever regret the two plus years I spent with my ex, the vacations, the engagement, the horrific breakup? Never. Because it opened me up to a new way of looking at dating. So did having cancer, believe it or not.

I think that when you're single and going through an illness like breast cancer, you learn more about your own body and what it needs than anyone will ever really understand. Somewhere along the way, the mental and the physical become aligned. While I used to be someone that looked for someone to always take care of me, I no longer felt I needed or wanted that. I knew that I could take care of myself, even when I was really at my lowest, and that experience made dating a lot different…at least it did for me. There was a lot less I was willing to put up with, particularly insecurities and idiosyncrasies that I no longer found "cute" or "endearing." As much as I decided that for the time being I didn't mind being single, my friends (who are all married, many with children) pleaded a different case.

"Just find someone cool we can hang out with, you owe us someone great," they complained.

I finally relented and started to take the whole online dating thing with a bigger grain of salt. I began taking my online dating process almost as seriously as I was taking my job search. The sheer awkwardness of meeting a total stranger face to face for the first time after exchanging snarky emails and text messages is enough to fill a novel. You always have a certain image in your head of what someone is going to look like and, in my experience, it's never right. For instance, one of my first dates, upon smiling, revealed a mouth of classic metal braces. Really?

My war stories about dating are, on the surface, no different from any other woman's plight to find the perfect guy. But the one question that you always get asked on a first date, especially in Washington DC, tended to lead me down a line of questioning that most people would warn never to talk about on a first date with a total stranger. For me this conversation was always make or break.

"So, what do you do?" they would ask as I slowly sipped on a glass of white wine.

"Well, I'm sort of a marketing consultant/writer," I'd explain. Sip, sip.

"Where do you work?"

"From home, at the moment."

And as most men would look at me quizzically, I would feel the instant need to reveal my big secret since there seems to be no way in hell that anyone that lives in Washington DC could possibly do anything other than work for the government.

"I'm actually looking for a job at the moment."

"Oh you got laid off?" A common question in 2011.

And it was usually at this point where I would share my tale of the past year. There was kind of no way of getting around it (though I think that many people would beg to differ). Why would I tell this acutely vulnerable story on a first date to a total stranger? Why would I talk about being diagnosed with breast cancer, of going through chemotherapy, radiation and freezing my hair? Well, to me, this story is who I am now, like it or not. It would come out sooner or later, so I figured why not get it out of the way sooner? Especially if the guy seemed like good news.

As I would share my tale with numerous dates, I always laughed because most people wouldn't believe me if I wasn't standing there talking about it. I had managed to turn my cancer into a one woman comedic tour, which was a coping mechanism I'm sure, but I constantly felt the need to assure my dates that I was 100% fine and would not keel over and spill my drink in their lap.

Once I told my story, almost every man that I've met since my diagnosis would immediately look down at my chest to see what I'm working with these days.

"They're real," I would respond to their downward gaze.

"Oh I wasn't…"

"Yes, you were, and it's OK."

Technically, I wasn't lying to these men. My breasts are real, but this point in the conversation typically let me know whether or not I was going to be ordering a second glass of wine. In addition to knowing that I was looking for someone who I'm compatible with, I also knew it was crucial to find someone who wasn't going to start looking at me like I am some kind of Make-A-Wish recipient. And sure, I received a variety of responses once I was done telling my story, but most men surprisingly made the cut. I remember one man in particular that responded to me by saying, "Wow, I should really play with my balls more." Actually.

Getting through any first date is tricky, but for me, it was what came after that was most confusing for me, especially considering that I was still a work in progress a year plus after surgery. I wasn't a year out of chemotherapy yet, meaning that I was still down one nipple since they don't replace it until you are a year out of chemo and radiation. In short, getting physical gave me way more anxiety than it ever had during my adult life. I had gotten used to having my breasts constantly examined by a slew of doctors, even if it was always a bit surreal. But having a lover do the same is a completely different story. There were those mid-make out session explanations I would give about why I wouldn't be completely topless, which were occasionally fueled by white wine. Typically, I'd then constantly replay the interaction in my mind, wondering whether or not I handled the situation well, and whether or not I'd ever see this person again. As much as I had spent the time working on myself and being secure in my new body, I had no control over what people I dated thought about it, and the lack of control was enough to drive me crazy. Sure, I was used to staring in the mirror at a mismatched top half, but no one else was obliged to do the same. They could move on and find someone who was complete.

There's one conversation that I had had in particular that will probably always stick with me. This guy made dating seem easy, like the way it should have always been. Not complicated. I like you, you like me; let's date and see what happens. Let's spend time together, and it just kind of was.

Sometime after three or four months of casually dating each other, I got a text from him: "So when do I get to see your boobs?" he asked. I told him that the right one was up for grabs whenever he wanted, but that, of course was not good enough (because why would it be for any man?). "Both or nothing," he replied. I tried to reiterate that my body was kind of a work in progress, to which he responded, "You think I'm going to judge you on a scar?" And the truth was simple: yes, I did. But how do you say that in a text message without sounding super insecure? In fact, I wasn't exactly insecure; it's not like I took a knife to myself and decided to carve up my body. This was the hand I was dealt. But there was still a part of me that didn't know how people would react, and that scared me. Sure, the guys that I dated knew right off the bat that I had cancer, but having that conversation is the easy part. Once I got that out of the way and determined whether or not they would be able just to handle that part, the technicalities of every other aspect came into play.

That day, I stared at the phone, trying to figure out how to answer. There was no response that made sense to me other than, "How about next time I just show you?" He agreed and I started to panic—that is, for a good ten minutes until I realized that it didn't matter. If he saw me topless and couldn't handle it, then you know what? He would never be worth my time.

Two weeks later, we found ourselves in my apartment, talking yet again about my boobs and I had to just "rip the band-aid off" and tell him the truth of what was being hidden underneath my $100 bras from Bloomies.

"Look, the right side, is totally normal, see," I said as I flashed him my right side. "My left side is a little, um, different." I paused to take a large sip of wine.

He looked at me, waiting for me to continue.

"I don't have a nipple. They take it away from you when you get reconstruction and I haven't exactly gotten it back yet."

His head cocked to the side for a minute and said, "Really?"

My stomach sunk a little. What would he do next? Would he put his glass of wine down and leave? Would he ask to see it? I really was kind of wandering into unchartered territory here and wasn't sure what was going to happen next.

"I'm going to tell you a story about when I was in the Army," he began and proceeded to tell me a pretty gruesome story about the Middle East and a gunshot victim that he had come across while over there.

"So, if you think that I'm going to judge you or not like you anymore because of a scar then you are fucking crazy."

I exhaled, not realizing that I had been holding my breath. "OK," I replied. "OK."

It was the perfect answer to an insanely scary conversation that I knew I'd eventually have to have when I found someone that was worth my time. Well, he was worth the conversation. It was at that point that I decided that I wanted to keep him around because a conversation like that does not always end well and this one did. But the good guys, the ones that are worth it, don't care because they already like you for who you are.

And that brings us to today.

It's been five years and five months since I heard the harrowing words, "I'm so sorry to tell you this, but you have cancer." It's been five years and four months since I underwent a seven hour surgery that radically changed the way I will look forever. It's been four years and nine months since I finished chemotherapy, which might have been the hardest thing I've ever gone through in my life. It's been four years and seven months since I finished radiation, leaving the left side of my chest raw for days. It's been three years and 10 months since I re-emerged myself into the real world and trying to reclaim the professional life that I once had.

I'm still here and I'm not going anywhere, whether anyone likes it or not.

I'm still here and I'm still laughing.

Works Cited

1. http://www.cancer.org/acs/groups/content/@epidemiologysurveilance/documents/document/acspc-030975.pdf
2. http://www.cancer.org/acs/groups/content/@epidemiologysurveilance/documents/document/acspc-030975.pdf
3. http://www.breastcancer.org/risk/factors/genetics.jsp
4. http://www.cancer.gov/cancertopics/factsheet/Risk/BRCA
5. http://www.cancer.org/acs/groups/content/@epidemiologysurveilance/documents/document/acspc-029771.pdf
6. http://www.mayoclinic.org/breast-cancer/tramsurgery.html
7. http://aboutcancer.com/chemotherapy_history.htm
8. http://my.clevelandclinic.org/services/pet_scan/hic_pet_scan.aspx
9. http://www.mayoclinic.com/health/ct-scan/MY00309
10. http://www.cancer.net/navigating-cancer-care/how-cancer-treated/chemotherapy/catheters-and-ports-cancer-treatment
11. http://chemocare.com/chemotherapy/drug-info/Taxotere.aspx
12. http://www.chemocare.com/bio/carboplatin.asp
13. http://m.herceptin.com/breast/adjuvant
14. https://penguincoldcaps.com/
15. http://www.mayoclinic.com/health/neutropenia/MY00110
16. http://www.cancer.org/treatment/treatmentsandsideeffects/physicalsideeffects/chemotherapyeffects/chemo-brain
17. http://www.cancercare.org/publications/70-coping_with_chemobrain_keeping_your_memory_sharp
18. http://www.medterms.com/script/main/art.asp?articlekey=3979
19. http://www.chemocare.com/managing/numbness__tingling.asp
20. https://disabilityrightslegalcenter.org/

Acknowledgment

This book. Oh this book. It started out of sheer boredom during one of my sleepless, steroid-infused evenings. "Maybe I should just write all of this down. Maybe I'll want to re-read this one day." And so it began. Little by little, cancer adventure after cancer adventure, I chronicled my illness through my final treatment and what comes after.

There were so many people in my corner that to this day, I have to stop and take a moment to reflect on just how lucky I am.

Team family: of course I would be nowhere without my parents. They schlepped from NY to DC every 21 days, sat with me for eight grueling hours, didn't flinch when I told them to fuck off and helped me reclaim my life once it was all over. I am their only child and I'm not always the easiest so for them I will always be eternally grateful.

To my cousin Barrie: who would have thought that our paths would have crossed in this way, but they did and your generosity essentially saved my sanity. By conserving my hair, it allowed me to walk down the street when I had the energy to without getting "that look" from strangers and to allow me to feel like a human being, rather than a science project. I will be forever thankful.

Team Friend: oh so many. All of you that called, texted, sent a card, checked in and generally just gave a shit; wow. I was always amazed at how lucky I was and continue to be grateful for all of you. My girls: Nic, JP, Dr. Tina, Sailagirl, Kath, Gooners. You all made me laugh when I needed to, vent when I needed to and drink obsessively when I needed to. The brothers I never asked for; Ricky and Mel and my forever roommate, Poolie.

To my roomies and family: Pleasance and Babby. When I look around whatever table we're sitting at; it's exactly how I thought it would be back in 728b. We will always go dancing and I will always be grateful for you both.

To Michie: from Kindergarten. KINDERGARTEN. Not many people can say that they've had the same best friend for over 30 years but I can and it's pretty unbelievable.

To J: thank you for making my post-cancer life exactly what I had hoped it would be; easy.

And to everyone that read my blog, posted something supportive, sent a funny text, made me laugh or cry (in a good way), thank you. They say that part of battling cancer is surrounding yourself with positivity and I am living proof that who you are around makes a difference. It's one of the reasons I'm still around to annoy you all today and for that, I have no more words.

About the Author

When Meredith Goldberg was three years old, she wanted to be a manicurist. Upon realizing that she lacked the artistic skill, she started making things up in her head including imaginary friends, which kept her company growing up as an only child on Long Island. Her imagination keeps running to this day where she is a Marketing Director in the hospitality industry. When diagnosed with breast cancer at the age of 32 and faced with a year of boredom, Goldberg began to chronicle her adventures with navigating this new world of doctors, medicine and what comes "next". Goldberg lives in Washington, DC where she spends her days eating, creating hashtags and dressing up Monti, her hotel's disaffected beagle. From Cocktails to Chemotherapy is her first non-fiction work.

Made in the USA
Columbia, SC
02 May 2017